# Special Format Serials and Issues:
## Annual Review of . . . ,
## Advances in . . . ,
## Symposia on . . . ,
## Methods in . . .

# Special Format Serials and Issues: Annual Review of ..., Advances in ..., Symposia on ..., Methods in ...

Tony Stankus

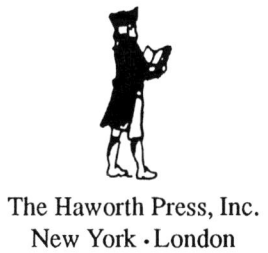

The Haworth Press, Inc.
New York ·London

*Special Format Serials and Issues: Annual Review of . . . , Advances in . . . , Symposia on . . . , Methods in . . .* has also been published as *The Serials Librarian*, Volume 27, Numbers 2/3 1995.

The Haworth Press, Inc., 10 Alice Street, Binghamton, NY 13904-1580 USA

### Library of Congress Cataloging-in-Publication Data

Stankus, Tony.
     Special format serials and issues: annual review of–, advances in–, symposia on–, methods in– / Tony Stankus.
        p. cm.
     Includes bibliographical references (p.    ) and index.
     ISBN 1-56024-799-1 (alk. paper)
     1. Science–Periodicals–Bibliography. 2. Engineering–Periodicals–Bibliography. I. Title.
Z7403.S8 1996
[QA1.A1]
016.505–dc20
                                      96-1022
                                         CIP

To Peter Perch

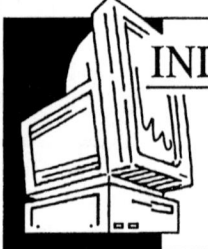

# INDEXING & ABSTRACTING

Contributions to this publication are selectively indexed or abstracted in print, electronic, online, or CD-ROM version(s) of the reference tools and information services listed below. This list is current as of the copyright date of this publication. See the end of this section for additional notes.

- *Academic Abstracts/CD-ROM,* EBSCO Publishing, P.O. Box 2250, Peabody, MA 01960-7250

- *Academic Search: database of 2,000 selected academic serials, updated monthly,* EBSCO Publishing, 83 Pine Street, Peabody, MA 01960

- *Cambridge Scientific Abstracts, Health & Safety Science Abstracts,* Environmental Routenet (accessed via INTERNET), 7200 Wisconsin Avenue, #601, Bethesda, MD 20814

- *Chemical Abstracts,* Chemical Abstracts Service Library, 2540 Olgentangy Road, P.O. Box 3012, Columbus, OH 43210

- *CINAHL (Cumulative Index to Nursing & Allied Health Literature), in print, also on CD-ROM from CD PLUS, EBSCO, and SilverPlatter, and online from CDP Online (fomerly BRS), Data-Star, and PaperChase. (Support materials include Subject Heading List, Database Search Guide, and instructional video.)* CINAHL Information Systems, P.O. Box 871, 1509 Wilson Terrace, Glendale, CA 91209-0871

- *CNPIEC Reference Guide: Chinese National Directory of Foreign Periodicals,* P.O. Box 88, Beijing, People's Republic of China

- *Current Awareness Bulletin,* Association for Information Management, Information House, 20-24 Old Street, London, EC1V 9AP, England

- *Current Contents* . . . . . see: *Institute for Scientific Information*

- *Hein's Legal Periodical Checklist: Index to Periodical Articles Pertaining to Law,* William S. Hein & Co., Inc., 1285 Main Street, Buffalo, NY 14209

- *IBZ International Bibliography of Periodical Literature,* Zeller Verlag GmbH & Co., P.O.B. 1949, d-49009 Osnabruck, Germany

- *Index to Periodical Articles Related to Law,* University of Texas, 727 East 26th Street, Austin, TX 78705

- *Information Reports & Bibliographies,* Science Associates International, Inc., 6 Hastings Road, Marlboro, NJ 07746-1313

(continued)

- *Information Science Abstracts,* Plenum Publishing Company, 233 Spring Street, New York, NY 10013-1578

- *Informed Librarian, The,* Infosources Publishing, 140 Norma Road, Teaneck, NJ 07666

- *Institute for Scientific Information,* 3501 Market Street, Philadelphia, Pennsylvania 19104. Coverage in:
  a) Social Science Citation Index (SSCI): print, online, CD-ROM
  b) Research Alerts (current awareness service)
  c) Social SciSearch (magnetic tape)
  d) Current Contents/Social & Behavioral Sciences (weekly current awareness service)

- *INTERNET ACCESS (& additional networks) Bulletin Board for Libraries ("BUBL"), coverage of information resources on INTERNET, JANET, and other networks.*
  - JANET X.29: UK.AC.BATH.BUBL or 00006012101300
  - TELNET: BUBL.BATH.AC.UK or 138.38.32.45 login 'bubl'
  - Gopher: BUBL.BATH.AC.UK (138.32.32.45). Port 7070
  - World Wide Web: http: / / www.bubl.bath.ac.uk./BUBL/ home.html
  - NISSWAIS: telnetniss.ac.uk (for the NISS gateway)
  The Andersonian Library, Curran Building, 101 St. James Road, Glasgow G4 ONS, Scotland

- *Konyvtari Figyelo-Library Review,* National Szechenyi Library, Centre for Library and Information Science, H-1827 Budapest, Hungary

- *Library & Information Science Abstracts (LISA),* Bowker-Saur Limited, Maypole House, Maypole Road, East Grinstead, West Sussex, RH19 1HH, England

- *Library Digest,* Highsmith Press, W5527 Highway 106, P.O. Box 800, Fort Atkinson, WI 53538-0800

- *Library Hi Tech News,* Pierian Press, P.O. Box 1808, Ann Arbor, MI 48106

- *Library Literature,* The H. W. Wilson Company, 950 University Avenue, Bronx, NY 10452

- *MasterFILE: updated database,* EBSCO Publishing, 83 Pine Street, Peabody, MA 01960

- *Newsletter of Library and Information Services,* China Sci-Tech Book Review, Library of Academia Sinica, 8 Kexueyuan Nanlu, Zhongguancun, Beijing 100080, People's Republic of China

- *PASCAL International Bibliography, T205: Sciences de l' information Documentation,* INIST/CNRS-Service Gestion des Documents Primaires, 2, allee du Parc de Brabois, F-54514 Vandoeuvre-les-Nancy, Cedex, France

(continued)

- *Periodica Islamica,* Berita Publishing, 22 Jalan Liku, 59100 Kuala Lumpur, Malaysia

- *Referativnyi Zhurnal (Abstracts Journal of the Institute of Scientific Information of the Republic of Russia),* The Institute of Scientific Information, Baltijskaja ul., 14, Moscow A-219, Republic of Russia

- *Social Science Citation Index . . . . see: Institute for Scientific Information*

- *Sociological Abstracts (SA),* Sociological Abstracts, Inc., P.O. Box 22206, San Diego, CA 92192-0206

## SPECIAL BIBLIOGRAPHIC NOTES

*related to special journal issues (separates)*
*and indexing/abstracting*

☐ indexing/abstracting services in this list will also cover material in any "separate" that is co-published simultaneously with Haworth's special thematic journal issue or DocuSerial. Indexing/abstracting usually covers material at the article/chapter level.

☐ monographic co-editions are intended for either non-subscribers or libraries which intend to purchase a second copy for their circulating collections.

☐ monographic co-editions are reported to all jobbers/wholesalers/approval plans. The source journal is listed as the "series" to assist the prevention of duplicate purchasing in the same manner utilized for books-in-series.

☐ to facilitate user/access services all indexing/abstracting services are encouraged to utilize the co-indexing entry note indicated at the bottom of the first page of each article/chapter/contribution.

☐ this is intended to assist a library user of any reference tool (whether print, electronic, online, or CD-ROM) to locate the monographic version if the library has purchased this version but not a subscription to the source journal.

☐ individual articles/chapters in any Haworth publication are also available through the Haworth Document Delivery Services (HDDS).

# Special Format Serials and Issues:
# Annual Review of . . . ,
# Advances in . . . ,
# Symposia on . . . ,
# Methods in . . .

## CONTENTS

# ABOUT THE AUTHOR

With the goal of building competence and confidence in the many nonscientists who find themselves in science library jobs, Tony Stankus has written over 40 research papers, chapters, bibliographic essays, and reviews. Along the same lines, he has also authored or edited the following Haworth Press books:

- *Scientific Journals: Issues in Library Selection and Management* 1987. ISBN: 0-86656-616-3.
- *Scientific Journals: Improving Library Collections Through Analysis of Publishing Trends,* 1990. ISBN: 0-86656-905-7.
- *Biographies of Scientists for Sci-Tech Libraries: Adding Faces to the Facts,* 1991. ISBN: 1-56024-214-0.
- *Making Sense of Journals in the Physical Sciences,* 1992. ISBN: 1-56024-180-2.
- *Making Sense of Journals in the Life Sciences,* 1992. ISBN: 1-56024-181-0.
- *Science Librarianship at America's Liberal Arts Colleges: Working Librarians Tell Their Stories,* 1992. ISBN: 1-56024-357-0.
- *Scientific and Clinical Literature for the Decade of the Brain,* 1993. ISBN: 1-56024-481-X.

Tony took his degrees from the College of the Holy Cross (*Summa Cum Laude*) and from the University of Rhode Island Graduate School of Library and Information Studies (Distinguished Alumnus Award, 1992). He has been Science Librarian at the first school since 1974 and an Adjunct Professor at the second since 1982. His wife of 17 years, Mary Frances, is an instructor at Quinsigamond Community College's Nursing Skills Laboratory. Husband and wife are both gardeners (she does flowers; he does vegetables). They are also lectors at St. Paul's Cathedral, the inner city church of the local Catholic diocese.

# Foreword

## THE DEMAND FOR REVIEWS

Students and faculty, scientists and physicians, and many others need review articles. In the first chapter of this work, Tony Stankus explains why review literature is heavily used and should be an important part of our collections. Yet, reviews can be overlooked because, undeniably, the primary focus of our library literature has been on building for our patrons collections that emphasize the reporting of original scientific, engineering, and medical results. We may overlook the need for the power of reviews to synthesize all of these fragmented reports.

There have been, however, improvements in our ability to find valuable reviews, particularly when they appear in journals that also feature original research articles. Consider the methods our patrons use to retrieve journal articles today. With the innovation and widespread availability of abstracting and indexing (A & I) tools on CD-ROM, utilization of journal literature is easier, in part, because it is so much faster to identify relevant articles, including reviews.

Let us take biomedicine as an example, an easy and pertinent choice for us, since half the chapters in this work involve biomedi-

---

Frank R. Kellerman has a BA from the University of Michigan and an MSLS from Case Western Reserve University. He is Biomedical Reference Librarian at Brown University's Sciences Library, and an adjunct professor at the Graduate School of Library and Information Studies at the University of Rhode Island where he teaches courses on Health Sciences Librarianship; Indexing and Abstracting; and Online Searching and Services.

[Haworth co-indexing entry note]: "Foreword." Kellerman, Frank R. Co-published simultaneously in *The Serials Librarian* (The Haworth Press, Inc.) Vol. 27, No. 2/3, 1995, pp. xiii-xxi; and: *Special Format Serials and Issues: Annual Review of . . . , Advances in . . . , Symposia on . . . , Methods in . . .* (ed: Tony Stankus) The Haworth Press, Inc., 1995, pp. xiii-xxi. Single or multiple copies of this article are available from The Haworth Document Delivery Service [1-800-342-9678, 9:00 a.m. - 5:00 p.m. (EST)].

*xiii*

cine. In 1988, the National Library of Medicine (NLM) made a major change in its method of indexing review papers. This served to expand the definition of review, showed an appreciation of the variety of reviews, and generally highlighted the importance of reviews. Before this, MEDLINE searchers could only use "review" to retrieve the traditional, fairly comprehensive review of the current research on a specific subject. Now searchers are encouraged by the new scheme to intentionally limit their searches by using an expanded variety of review categories.[1-3] Compare search results under the old system (13,800 reviews in 1987) with the more sophisticated categorization now:

- Review, Academic–the traditional, fairly comprehensive review of current research on a specific subject
  4,084
- Review, Tutorial–a broad introduction to a field for a student or an update for a physician
  30,651
- Review, Multicase–each article reviews hundreds of cases and may be most useful for epidemiologists
  727
- Review of Reported Cases–reports on a case(s) with a review of earlier cases
  3,159
- Review Literature–this is a general term for reviews that do not fit into other categories
  1,378
- Review–to retrieve all review articles regardless of specific type, use this publication type code. It is assigned to all review articles
  40,192

The 1994 total of 40,192 represents a remarkable rise. Part of this may be an increase in the actual number of reviews, but most of it is from the enhanced capacity of the systems in identifying reviews. (Note that adding together the numbers from the specific types does not equal the total. An individual article may be assigned more than one of the specific review types. Also, not all review types are listed in this breakdown.) Moreover, a better and confirming appreciation of the rising importance of reviews can be had through a look at the database as a whole. In the last year of the old indexing system, less than 5% of the articles were indexed as reviews. In 1994, the proportion was over 10%.[4]

Intriguingly, the national debate on health care reform is also connected to the revised indexing of review literature. Indexers started assigning the publication type, Meta-Analysis, in 1993. Meta-Analyses utilize quantitative methods on the results derived from many previously published studies so as to come up with a statistically-based policy position paper. For example, a meta-analysis may take and combine the data contained in several different colon cancer clinical trials so as to evaluate the effectiveness of competing therapies. This combination, comparison, and meta-analytic integration then enables planners to come to more robust and certain guidelines. While meta-analyses are not indexed as reviews, they certainly are designed for the same purpose: the synthesizing of the main points of key literature for scientists and physicians.

## THE RANKING AND PRICES OF REVIEW JOURNALS

*Journal Citation Reports* (JCR) provides a number of rankings of serials that are covered by *Science Citation Index*. A look at the key method of ranking journals, a per-paper-per-year approximation called the "Impact Factor," provides more evidence of the importance of review papers and of the serials that carry these reviews. Consider the following example from the 1991 *Reports*. Out of the 4,292 journals ranked by impact factor, these are the top ten:[5]

| | | |
|---|---|---|
| 1. | *Clinical Research* | 37.160 |
| 2. | * *Annual Review of Biochemistry* | 35.552 |
| 3. | * *Annual Review of Immunology* | 33.962 |
| 4. | *Cell* | 30.247 |
| 5. | * *Annual Review of Cell Biology* | 23.641 |
| 6. | * *Microbiological Reviews* | 23.250 |
| 7. | *New England Journal of Medicine* | 23.223 |
| 8. | * *Advances in Nuclear Physics* | 20.000 |
| 9. | * *Pharmacological Reviews* | 20.000 |
| 10. | *Science* | 19.607 |

Note the six titles with asterisks in this list. These are serials specifically devoted to reviews alone, a remarkable showing. What is almost as impressive is that all four remaining titles also feature intermittent reviews. There is more good news about review serials: a number of them are among the most reasonable titles in their disciplines. Note, for example, in the previous list, the presence of a number of members of the Annual Reviews family. This impact leadership is no fluke[6] and is happily coupled with affordability right down the line. Consider this table of 1994 prices:

| | |
|---|---|
| *Annual Review of Astronomy and Astrophysics* | *$60* |
| *Annual Review of Biochemistry* | *$49* |
| *Annual Review of Cell Biology* | *$46* |
| *Annual Review of Earth and Planetary Sciences* | *$62* |
| *Annual Review of Ecology and Systematics* | *$47* |
| *Annual Review of Fluid Mechanics* | *$47* |
| *Annual Review of Immunology* | *$48* |
| *Annual Review of Materials Science* | *$75* |
| *Annual Review of Microbiology* | *$48* |
| *Annual Review of Neuroscience* | *$48* |
| *Annual Review of Nuclear and Particle Science* | *$62* |

Compare those to the average price of the journals of the specialties. Here is a sample from a study of titles and prices of journals covered by *Index Medicus* in 1992:[7]

| | | |
|---|---|---|
| Allergy and Immunology | 82 titles | average price $380. |
| Biochemistry | 66 titles | average price $970. |
| Cytology | 55 titles | average price $440. |
| Microbiology | 61 titles | average price $352. |
| Neurosciences | 22 titles | average price $793. |

In summary, reviews and review serials are worth knowing better because:

- they are easier to retrieve through A & I services than ever before and will be more likely to be demanded by patrons.
- scientists clearly cite them disproportionately.
- they include some of the best bargains in scientific literature.

## PUBLISHED SYMPOSIA

Symposia proceedings take a lot of abuse from librarians. We often see them as expensive, often unrefereed, and published too long after the actual meeting. From our point of view, these would seem to be the best candidates for migration to a largely electronic form of distribution, perhaps for free on the Internet. There may be another side to the story. There is scarcely a major scientific, clinical, or technical society that does not continue to hold these meetings, and issue some print documentation of their content. Meetings may be large or small. They may cover a broad discipline with thousands of attendees or focus on a specific problem with a few experts. A search of MEDLINE, for example, shows that between 1990-1994, there were 1,032 Consensus Development Conferences in print, 212 from the prestigious National Institutes of Health alone.[8] If anything, the number of symposia in print grows and those symposia have their own A & I service, *Index to Scientific & Technical Proceedings* (ISTP). The following table represents the numbers of symposia ISTP has covered for given years.[9]

| | |
|------|-------|
| 1984 | 3,358 |
| 1986 | 3,957 |
| 1988 | 4,074 |
| 1990 | 4,186 |
| 1992 | 4,167 |
| 1994 | 4,218 |

How are these conferences reported in print? Are some, like some review papers, mingled among regular papers in journals one takes already? The answer is yes. In 1994, 2,055 were published as part of regular subscriptions to journals, about half the overall total. Where did the remaining half, 2,163, appear? The answer is in what is often called a monographic series, but is more properly termed a continuation. Consider the following table of titles with the number of volumes indexed in 1994.

*Proceedings of the Society of Photo-Optical Instrumentation Engineers (SPIE)* 287

These are among the best known, and are characterized by multiple volumes each year. To add to this complication is the issue of price. Whereas review series are worth knowing partly because they contain many bargains, continuations based on symposia are worth watching because their prices can be quite high. It is not unusual for each symposium volume in a continuation to cost over $100. The average price for a title in the *AIP Conference Proceedings* listed above is $150. You will need to become familiar with their patterns of publication. Are you being charged for volumes that did not come? The alternative is to buy them as individual books and not have these publications come on continuation. Tony Stankus explains what to look for–which publications in each discipline deliver good value.

### METHODS PAPERS

The title of an editorial in *The Scientist*, a newspaper from the Institute for Scientific Information, gives a hint to the role of the methods papers in science: "The 4 Most Cited Papers–Magic in These Methods."[10] Columns and articles and notes that report on the "Most-Cited Papers of All Time" show methodology papers at the top. The all time leader is a 1951 article on protein determination by Oliver H. Lowry. Through 1988 it had been cited 187,652 times and in 1988 alone was cited by 9,750 papers.[11] Why are methods papers so heavily cited? From Lowry, talking modestly about his paper's citation record: "It just happened to be a trifle better or easier or more sensitive than other methods, and of course nearly everyone measures protein these days."[12]

Methods are useful. Tony Stankus goes further in analyzing their role. One of the reasons that he discusses comes from the structure of the original research article itself. The methodology part is always carefully given its own section heading in the paper, but the methods themselves are not fully described. The citation to the original methods paper serves two purposes. It gives credit to the technique being used and it also saves space in the journal issue. Journal editors often allow fewer pages for the paper than the author may wish.

*Methods in Enzymology* is a premier methods serial. It began in 1955 and during 1995 hit its 250th volume. Each volume brings together papers on methods centered around a specific topic, e.g., v.193, *Mass Spectrometry*. From 1972 through 1994 there were 9,962 papers from it indexed in MEDLINE. As determined through the *Science Citation Index*, one of the most cited papers in history is Maxam, A. M. and Gilbert, W. "Sequencing End-Labeled DNA with Base-Specific Chemical Cleavages." *Methods in Enzymology* 65:499-560, 1980. In 1994 alone, there were 382 citations to this article. Here is a list of some of the journals containing articles citing that individual paper along with the number of citations to it:

- *Journal of Biological Chemistry*   59
- *Nucleic Acids Research*   34
- *Molecular and Cellular Biology*   26
- *Journal of Molecular Biology*   18
- *Biochemistry*   17
- *Journal of Bacteriology*   12
- *Journal of Virology*   11

The preceding examples have centered on the biomedical realm and have shortchanged the physical sciences which are also well covered in this book. Chemistry journals and reference materials are frequently among the most expensive, but are also heavily used. Although the Lowry paper was the extreme example, methods papers, it should be noted, may be used for quite some time by chemists. *Organic Syntheses* is a methods serial. One bound volume comes out per year containing about thirty methods papers at the modest price of about $45. Its subtitle is *An Annual Publication of Satisfactory Methods for the Preparation of Organic Chemicals*. Its standing with chemists goes beyond "satisfactory" and Stankus will describe its status. The chart below comes from the citing record to ten of the twenty-nine papers published in v.63, 1985. Note that in *Science Citation Index* several of these papers were cited varyingly as v.63, 1985 and also as v.63, 1984. The cited page numbers were the same, so for the purposes of this tally, they are counted as the same papers. Other citing discrepancies were not searched for. What is noteworthy here is the staying power of methods papers through the years. Citing in the first three years is similar to the citing level in years seven through nine.

| First Author and Page | '86 | '87 | '88 | '92 | '93 | '94 |
|---|---|---|---|---|---|---|
| Seebach D, p. 1 | 9 | 9 | 11 | 6 | 10 | 8 |
| Hajos ZG, p. 26 | 1 | 2 | 2 | 3 | 3 | 1 |
| Hill JG, p. 66 | 8 | 9 | 6 | 4 | 8 | 5 |
| Young SD, p. 79 | 1 | 1 | 2 | 0 | 1 | 1 |
| Seebach D, p. 109 | 4 | 2 | 0 | 1 | 1 | 0 |
| Ellis MK, p. 140 | 3 | 2 | 2 | 1 | 3 | 1 |
| Salaun J, p. 147 | 1 | 1 | 1 | 3 | 1 | 2 |
| Keller O, p. 160 | 2 | 4 | 1 | 7 | 6 | 0 |
| Shono T, p. 206 | 1 | 2 | 2 | 0 | 3 | 8 |
| Batcho AD, p. 214 | 3 | 1 | 1 | 2 | 0 | 0 |

This recitation of citation numbers and prices and indexing practices only serves as an antiseptic warmup to the topic at hand. Tony Stankus launches with chapter one a thorough and lively introduction to the nature of these three publication types. He discloses which materials our patrons depend on and why. After that introduction comes a discipline by discipline insightful account of the specific reviews, meetings, and methods serials. Above, *Organic Syntheses* was presented accompanied by a rather dry example. Stankus, in his knowledgeable and entertaining style, elevates the discussion to a clever mixture of peoples, publications, and science. Tony Stankus knows sciences serials. He is the expert and he writes about them in an engaging and entertaining style you will not find anywhere else.

*Frank R. Kellerman*

# REFERENCE NOTES

1. "Publication Types," in *Medical Subject Headings–Annotated Alphabetic List, 1995.* Bethesda, MD, National Library of Medicine, 1994, pp. I-18–I-26.

2. Snow, Bonnie. "Review Articles in MEDLINE: Past and Present," *Online* 13, no. 2 (March 1989):101-105.

3. "Review Literature," *NLM Technical Bulletin* (March 1988 Supplement no. 1):31-32.

4. "New Review Indexing Policy–Results One Year Later," *NLM Technical Bulletin* (February 1989 Supplement no.1):42.

5. *Journal Citation Reports; A Bibliometric Analysis of Science Journals in the ISI Database, 1991.* Philadelphia, Institute for Scientific Information, 1992, p. 7.

6. Woodward, A. M. and Hensman, Sandy. "Citations to Review Serials," *Journal of Documentation* 32, no. 4 (December 1976):290-293.

7. Fortney, Lynn M. and Basile, Victor A. *Index Medicus Price Study, 1988-1992.* Birmingham, AL, EBSCO, 1992.

8. "Publication Types," In *Medical Subject Headings–Annotated Alphabetic List, 1995.* Bethesda, MD, National Library of Medicine, 1994, pp. I-19.

9. *Index to Scientific & Technical Proceedings.* Philadelphia, Institute for Scientific Information, 1994, pp. 18A-19A.

10. Pendlebury, D. "The 4 Most Cited Papers–Magic in These Methods," *The Scientist* 2, no. 15 (1988):15.

11. Garfield, Eugene. "The Most-Cited Papers of All Time, SCI 1945-1988. Part 1A. The SCI Top 100–Will the Lowry Method Ever Be Obliterated?" *Essays of an Information Scientist* 13 (1990):45-56.

12. Garfield, Eugene. *Citation Indexing–Its Theory and Application in Science, Technology, and Humanities.* New York, Wiley, 1979. p. 246.

# Acknowledgments

*Joel Villa*, Coordinator of Audio-Visual Services, College of the Holy Cross, with both skill and courtesy, turned the tabular data originally intended for the Introduction into the reader-friendly graphs you now see.

*Lisa Sacovitch*, Assistant to the Science Librarian, College of the Holy Cross, used her considerable organizing skills to keep track of the many differing "editions" of each of these chapters, enabling the author to finally send to production only the most up-to-date revisions humanly possible.

*Frank Kellerman*, Brown University Sciences Library, wrote the Foreword, giving the reader a much better start than I could ever have provided. This is not a surprise. He's a lot smarter, but happened to be writing another book at the time!

# An Introduction to Three Special Genres Among Scientific Serials: Reviews, Symposia, and Methods

## THE SOMETIMES TROUBLING CHARACTERISTICS OF REVIEW AND SYMPOSIA SERIALS

There are many reasons why even rather capable serials and science librarians might have limited knowledge and even less regard of review journals, and of their cousins, symposia and theme issue serials, in the sciences. Probably the first is the general lack of uniformity of these special genres. It can be hard to see what a hardbound volume that calls itself a review (or symposium) that comes out about every third year has in common with a journal-like softbound monthly that also calls itself a review (or symposium). In many technical services departments, the first item would be handled as a "continuation" (handled with equal probability by monographic acquisitions or by periodicals) while the second would almost certainly be handled by the periodicals people. Rational expectations of where these items might be shelved in any given library are often frustrated. The same series is among the circulating monographs in one institution, among the noncirculating bound periodicals in a second, and, particularly if it is fat and irregular, treated as a kind of bibliography in the reference collection of a third.

The publication histories of some special genre serials resemble soap operas in their many plot twists and turns. One might start with

[Haworth co-indexing entry note]: "An Introduction to Three Special Genres Among Scientific Serials: Reviews, Symposia, and Methods." Stankus, Tony. Co-published simultaneously in *The Serials Librarian* (The Haworth Press, Inc.) Vol. 27, No. 2/3, 1995, pp. 1-37; and: *Special Format Serials and Issues: Annual Review of . . . , Advances in . . . , Symposia on . . . , Methods in . . .* (ed: Tony Stankus) The Haworth Press, Inc., 1995, pp. 1-37. Single or multiple copies of this article are available from The Haworth Document Delivery Service [1-800-342-9678, 9:00 a.m. - 5:00 p.m. (EST)].

a planned sequence of four books in a broadly defined subject area, each with its own author, title, and ISBN, if also with publisher-assigned series number. Suddenly and somewhat mysteriously, the next number becomes a collection of talks given at a conference, is proclaimed "volume five," and gets invoiced through a subscription agent. It might continue in this vein until volume eight, when it just as suddenly becomes a softbound quarterly. This might continue until diminished manuscript flow, some financial squeeze, or even an intentional "tenth anniversary combined issue," seems to give the publisher the idea of a hardcover annual!

Review serials and their relatives also present financial dilemmas for librarians. Not only do their prices rise as inexorably as other more "regular" science journals, but some publishers market "special issues" as both a serial and a monograph, so that it is entirely possible that overworked librarians may end up paying for two copies when only one was wanted, and feel duped in the process. Still other journal watchers feel that publishers are either diluting the percentage of peer-reviewed papers or padding an already overpriced bill with special issues that exclusively feature reviews or are dedicated to symposia.

The author, as a working science librarian, sees much validity in the complaints of his colleagues, and has experienced his share of confusion with these special genres. Nonetheless, the guiding principle of this book is a focus on what these serials try to do for their scientific audiences, not what they do to the equilibrium of the librarians who handle them. Along the way, the reader of this book hopefully will learn about the many types of scientific reviews as well as the differing degrees to which scientific conferences are archived in print. The diversity of formats that we see today can be better understood, if not exactly celebrated, by a look at the publishing traditions of given scientific fields and the role of competition between publishers, whether not-for-profit or commercial.

This author's ranking of competing special genre serials in this book is more experiential than purely citation-data-driven, for a variety of reasons. While it is clear to this author that "impact factors" in the annual installments of *Journal Citation Reports* from the Institute for Scientific Information can often provide useful insights when evaluating journals that are closely matched by subject and purpose, many irregular serials tend not to have "impact factors" reported. (ISI treats them like many fine technical services librarians do, as monographic series, and those do not get *JCR* impact factors.) Moreover, many other review serials do not really match their apparent competition because they have a differing underlying mission than other review sources in the same subject field. (For example, they might stress tutorial reviews as opposed to reviews for advanced researchers.) Using the impact factors that are available in these comparisons could still be unfair. In these and many other cases, the reader is better served by an explanation of the differing strategies and niches of these publications, as found through this author's direct examination. While this author, in weighing the relative value of competitors, remains influenced by citation data whenever appropriate, and is very mindful of the relative costs of competing special genre journals, specific impact factors and prices are not reported. These can be readily checked with greater currency in appropriate sources, such as the above cited *JCR*'s and most subscription agency and publisher catalogs. Nor is this work intended to be a substitute for other sources that enable one to find individual papers, issues or volumes of review or symposia. The *Index to Scientific Reviews*, the *Index to Scientific and Technical Proceedings*, *Proceedings in Print,* and many discipline-specific indexing and abstracting services do that job very well. To their credit, serially issued directories, both in print and on disc, are also likely to have many more entries than this work. However, exhaustive lists such as those have practical limitations in the three tasks that this author has set for himself. These are: gently orienting the reader, showing how the publications fit together, and helping the reader make choices in libraries with only limited funds. This book is about better understanding the hundreds of special genre serials one is most likely to consider in the majority of libraries, not about the thousands that conceivably could be run to ground by libraries with many millions of volumes and dollars in the now quixotic quest to become archives of record. This work nonetheless surveys a wide variety of scientific disciplines with a view to those who are considering their ongoing continuance or cancellation. We discuss not only those publications that are exclusively devoted to reviews or symposia (or later on, methods), but note some of the more important regular journals that undertake this work from time to time. In some cases, librarians will view those double-duty journals as having added (or sometimes diminished) value, and this too may sway decisions concerning their collection management. Moreover, in some fields, the paucity or absence of special genre journals can be best explained by the fact that a given society or publisher has decided to handle their functions within these more general journals.

Each subject chapter contains an abbreviated lay-level introduction to the field discussed. These describe the scope of topics covered, and foreshadow for those without specialty backgrounds, how some terminologically unfamiliar titles fit into the discussion. There is a distinct effort made at setting priorities, usually on a three-tier scheme, with the most essential items suggested for even small collections, with information on other titles provided for medium and large institutions that can collect somewhat more comprehensively.

## THE SCIENTIST'S NEED FOR A PANORAMA IN A WORLD OF SNAPSHOTS: THE ROLE OF A REVIEW

Each year, more and more articles describing small pieces of scientific research appear. In what some librarians regard as an effort to multiply the number of entries in their resumes, scientific authors break what might have been a single meaningful paper into as many "least-publishable-units" as possible. These can include several trial-balloon convention abstracts, and up to a dozen brief communications of preliminary findings.

But there is little incentive for scientific authors to heed librarian critics. Studies by librarians themselves have shown that "letters journals"–publishing vehicles specifically designed for brief preliminary works–are habitually among the most cited of journals. Consider the case of the *Proceedings of the National Academy of Sciences*. Election to the Academy is the highest honor for a U.S. scientist short of the Nobel Prize. With election comes the virtually absolute right to publish in this prestigious journal, effectively subject to one important rule: no paper there can exceed five pages! The "letters" phenomenon has given rise to many other journals specifically limited to short papers. Indeed, in many cases the letters offshoots of a full-length journal are demonstrably more cited than their parent publications (see Figure 1). Scientists argue that the need for speed of dissemination of results, and the need to repeatedly indicate progress in ongoing work to the granting agencies that are funding it are more reasonable explanations for their behavior than those posited by librarians. There is also some evidence–the Nobel Prizewinning paper of less than a full page length by Watson and Crick proposing a structure for DNA being a good example–that especially among scientists, the soul of wit is indeed brevity. But the problem with the majority of such cases of scientific wit is that they are increasingly becoming a kind of "inside joke," which fewer and fewer people, including many within the same specialty, "get" anymore. The audiences lack the context to make the stories work. In an era of increasing electronic journals, where article length is often only a few "screens," the multiplication of isolated bits of knowledge is increasing exponentially. We have more information than ever, and arguably less perspective on it than ever before.

Is there any hope for compensating for this atomization of important scientific announcements? One answer has actually been known for some time: it lies in review papers, and in the serials that particularly emphasize them. In review papers the author researches the research papers of many other authors. He or she provides answers to questions such as: What is the source for an idea? What motivates continued research on it? How much has already been done? How does it fit together? Are all the papers equally important? Which papers support an idea? Which contradict it? What seems to be resolved? What remains to be done? What has this research movement learned from other specialty efforts? What does it teach other specialties? Is this a good time to enter this field? Largely because reviews have answered these questions so well, many review journals are the most cited journals in their specialty, beating out even "letters" journals (see Figure 2). While there are other ways of providing a sense of scientific perspective through serials, the review journal is clearly the dominant approach in science and is the primary focus of this book. The numbers (now in the hundreds) and costs of review serials (also now in the hundreds) demand the attention of

FIGURE 1. Impact factors favor "letters" journals with many brief papers having little contextual discussion over traditional full-length papers that provide some background.

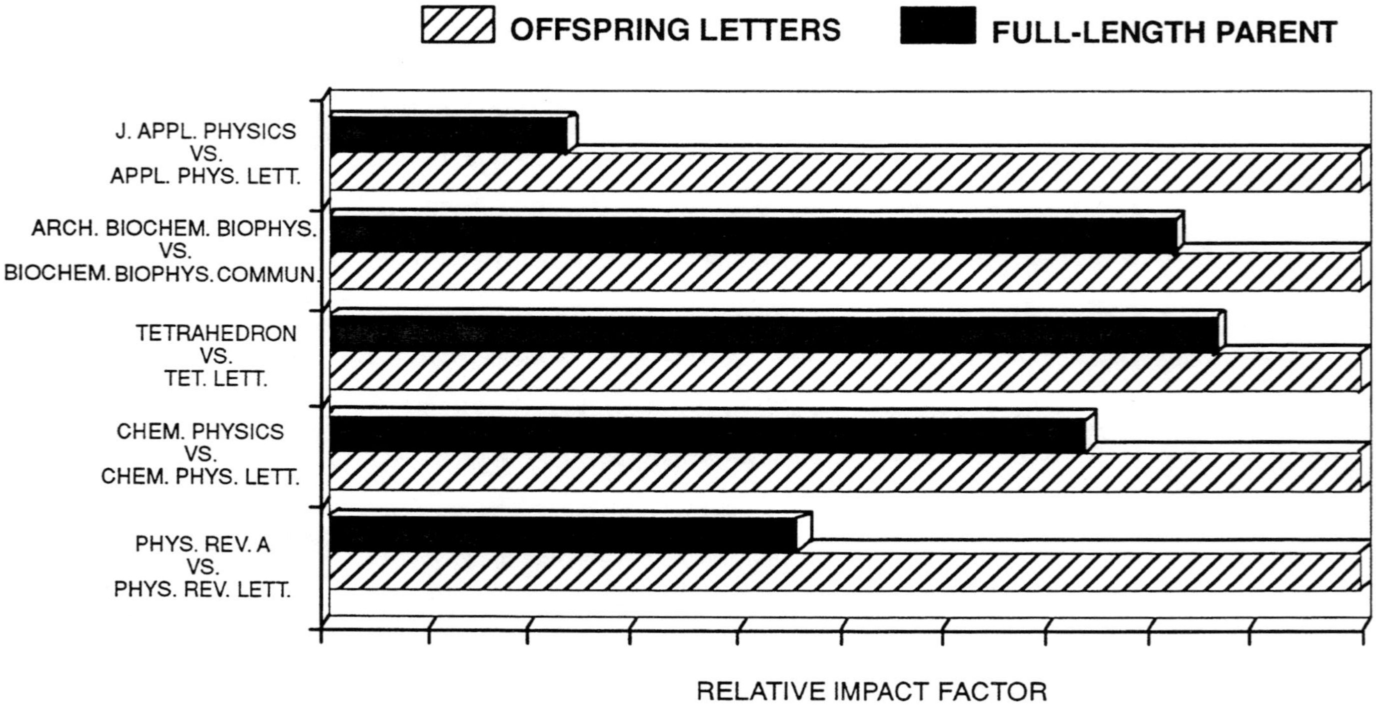

OFFSPRING LETTERS     FULL-LENGTH PARENT

J. APPL. PHYSICS
VS.
APPL. PHYS. LETT.

ARCH. BIOCHEM. BIOPHYS.
VS.
BIOCHEM. BIOPHYS. COMMUN.

TETRAHEDRON
VS.
TET. LETT.

CHEM. PHYSICS
VS.
CHEM. PHYS. LETT.

PHYS. REV. A
VS.
PHYS. REV. LETT.

RELATIVE IMPACT FACTOR

FIGURE 2. But review serials which are characterized by extensive discussion and contextual integration are more often cited than even "letters" journals.

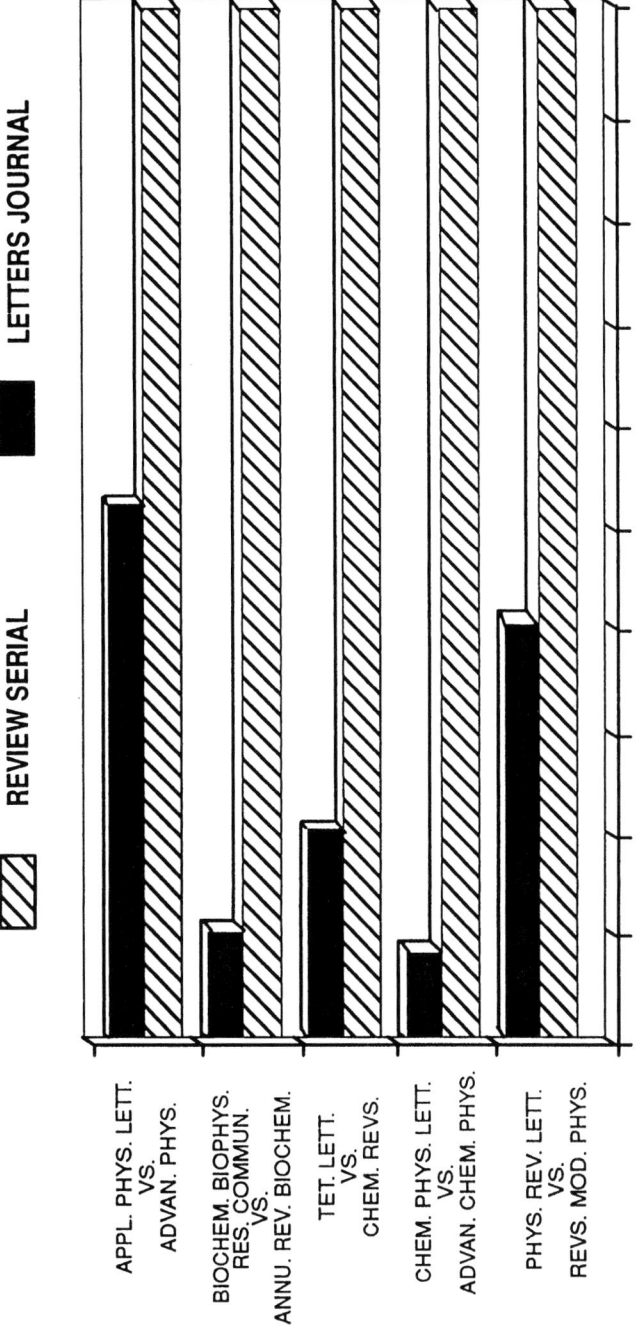

RELATIVE IMPACT FACTOR

today's collection managers seeking to provide their readers with what amounts to the essence of scientific progress.

## *WHO WRITES REVIEWS?*

Examination of the editorial policy of most journals that regularly publish reviews, particularly those devoted solely to reviews, clearly indicates that most of their authors are specifically invited to write them by the editors. In a small number of cases, *ideas* for a review are allowed to be submitted by any potential author. The author is, however, cautioned that he or she might well have to wait for an investigation by the editors of the desirability of such a review, as well as his or her fitness to write it. This seemingly antidemocratic approach has its roots in the power vested in review papers as documents of historical perspective, controversy evaluation, and agenda-setting. Because judgements of inclusion and exclusion of given scientific developments are very often involved in review writing, the doubts that a reader may entertain concerning the qualifications of an author to make these decisions must be addressed quickly and decisively. Editors deliberately seek out as authors those researchers with a long record of their own contributions to a field. They want people whose very name is synonymous with work in the specialty. This is bolstered when the author is affiliated with a research center known more generally for work in this area. Moreover, it is expected that the invited author has already developed a working familiarity through his or her own diligent reading of many of the major papers that could be discussed in the review, and has ready access through an excellent library to any others that might crop up along the way.

Despite this checklist of qualifications demanded of authors, and the entrenched advantages thought to be accrued by them, there are still complaints from both the writers and readers of reviews. One of the principal concerns of authors is the time involved to write a conscientious review. Who will continue to run their labs and write their papers while they examine everyone else's work? The earnest nominee for review authorship has often built up such an astounding record of publishing original research articles because his or her employer demanded it or the individual's personal compulsion has driven them to it–and those circumstances or demons may be hard to change. One of the more curious phenomena involving reviews is that while regular articles frequently involve not only the laboratory's senior scientist but his colleagues, post-doc's, graduate students, and technicians, most reviews have only one or two coauthors (see Figure 3). Once again, editors tend to discourage too many coauthors so as not to dim the canonical halo of the hand-picked author. The silent partner on most review papers is more likely to be a librarian who will serve the nominee through searching, assembling, and rechecking the pertinent papers and references. Finally, apart from a certain measure of prestige, there is often no reward for this sustained labor. Some for-profit publishers do pay an honorarium of a few hundred dollars, but this is modest compensation considering that most of these authors must carefully administer laboratory budgets and grants in the hundreds of thousands of dollars annually. One of the few perquisites is that authors who have done a good job in one year are often invited to sit on the editorial board in the next, so as to visit this "honor" on other, unsuspecting researchers in turn. Critics suggest that this phenomenon is akin to the propensity of abused children to become child abusers later in life.

Yet another complaint from review authors is that review papers, which often contain critical remarks, make as many enemies as friends. The enemies are most commonly of two types: those who feel their work was ignored; those who feel their work was noted but misunderstood or underemphasized. A less frequent third type might be those who feel they could have done a better job, with a fourth who argue that the topic surveyed by the author was secondary to one he or she would have preferred. (Never mind that it is generally the editors who designate the topic.)

Readers, particularly those at smaller institutions or from Third World countries, can also argue that the cozy relationship of editors and authors leads to a kind of hegemony of relatively few scholars, few institutions, and few nationalities represented in the leading review serials. This is often readily demonstrable (see Figures 4 and 5). The answer of review editors is that people of sufficient insight and commitment have always been scarce, and that prestigious schools and wealthier nations have made it a point to recruit them energeti-

FIGURE 3. Authorship of reviews is often still a personal burden in an age of long coauthor lists for regular articles.

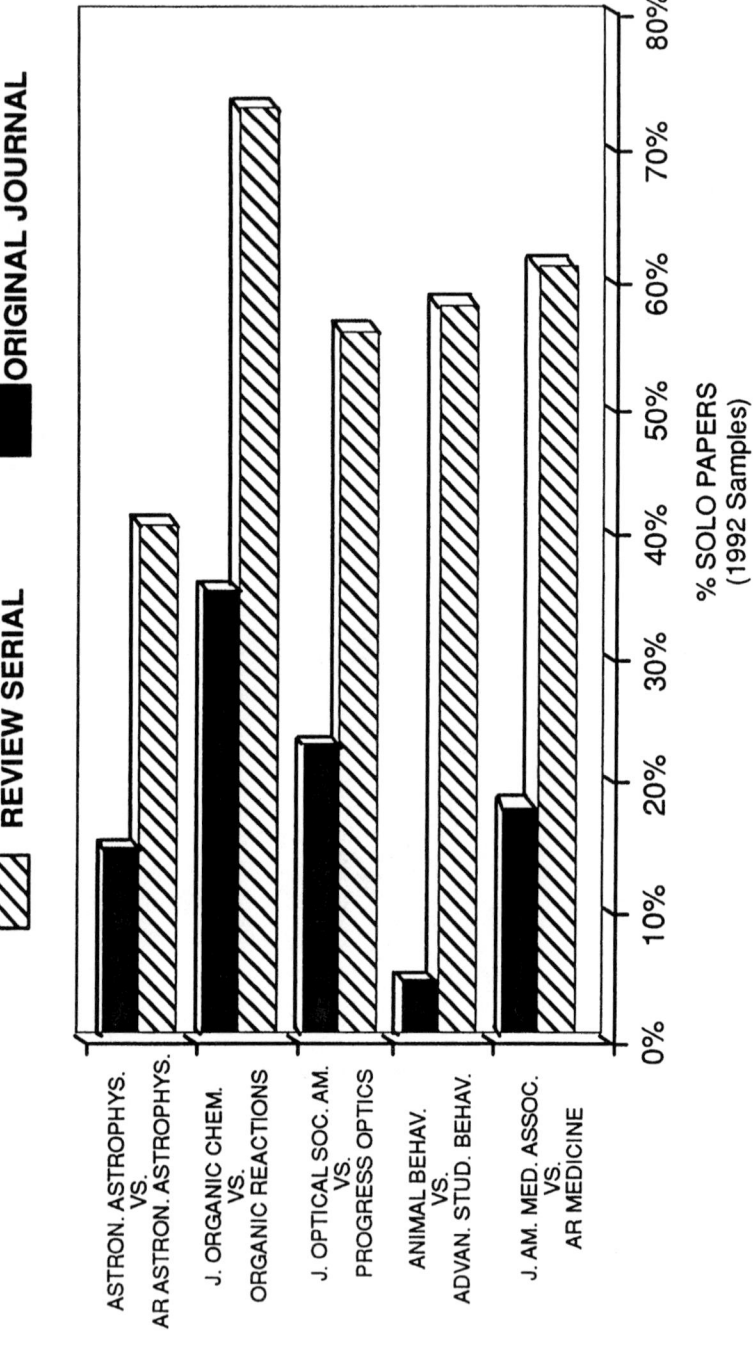

FIGURE 4. While critics argue that U.S. authors dominate leading reviews decade after decade, the U.S. has dominated Nobel Prizes in subject areas matching those reviews, a kind of vindication.

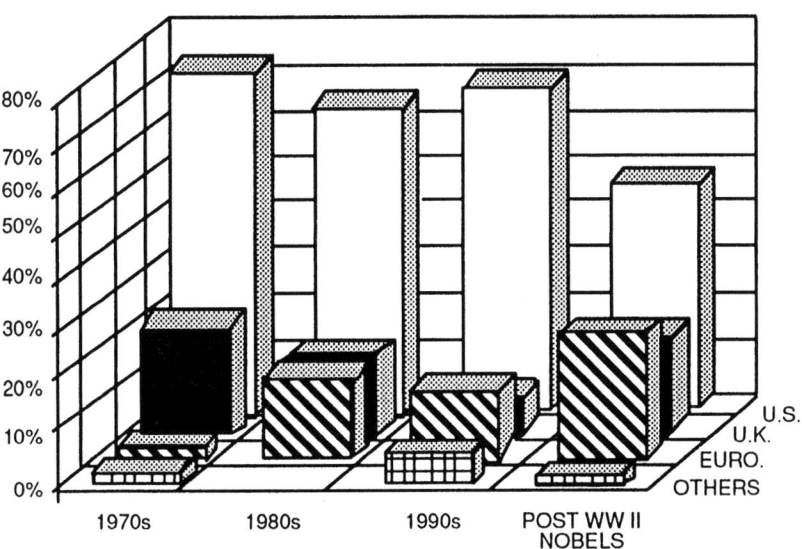

cally. Editors note that it is really a case of recruited scholars continuing to make the same narrow assortment of schools great year after year, not some sort of osmosis effect of the institutions on the leading scholars. (Parents of dull children, who pay hefty tuitions in the hopes of having something sink into those children from the academic atmosphere are, of course, told the osmosis story and thankfully believe it.) Review editors keep going to the same top institutions for review authors using the same sort of logic Great Depression-era folk heroes Bonnie and Clyde recounted to a reporter when asked why they repeatedly robbed banks: "because that's where the money is!"

## *WHERE ARE REVIEW PAPERS TO BE FOUND? FROM EXILE TO A PLACE OF THEIR OWN*

Historically, many British and American society-sponsored journals included review papers as a regular feature alongside regular

FIGURE 5. While critics argue that the same schools dominate reviews decade after decade, those same schools also dominate U.S. Nobel Prizes, a kind of vindication (from selected Annual Reviews).

| 1970s 10% UNIVS. YIELD 76% REVIEWS (ALPHABETICALLY) | 1980s 10% UNIVS. YIELD 69% REVIEWS (ALPHABETICALLY) | 1990s 10% UNIVS. YIELD 67% REVIEWS (ALPHABETICALLY) | NOBEL PRIZE UNIVERSITIES 10% UNIVS. YIELD 93% PRIZES (ALPHABETICALLY) |
| --- | --- | --- | --- |
| CALTECH* | ARIZONA | ARIZONA | BROWN |
| CHICAGO* | CALTECH* | CALTECH* | CALTECH* |
| COLORADO | CHAPEL HILL | CHAPEL HILL | CHICAGO* |
| HARVARD* | CHICAGO* | COLUMBIA | COLUMBIA* |
| ILLINOIS* | DUKE | DUKE | CORNELL |
| JOHNS HOPKINS* | HARVARD* | HARVARD* | HARVARD* |
| MINNESOTA | ILLINOIS* | ILLINOIS* | ILLINOIS* |
| PENN* | JOHNS HOPKINS* | JOHNS HOPKINS* | JOHNS HOPKINS* |
| ROCKEFELLER* | MARYLAND | MICHIGAN* | MICHIGAN* |
| STANFORD* | MINNESOTA | MINNESOTA | M.I.T.* |
| SUNY BUFFALO | M.I.T.* | PRINCETON | PENN* |
| TEXAS* | STANFORD* | ROCHESTER | PRINCETON* |
| U.C. BERKELEY* | SUNY BUFFALO | STANFORD* | ROCHESTER* |
| U.C.L.A. | TEXAS | U.C. BERKELEY* | ROCKEFELLER* |
| U.C. SAN DIEGO | U.C. BERKELEY* | U.C.L.A. | STANFORD* |
| U.C. SAN FRAN. | U.C.L.A. | U.C. SAN DIEGO | TEXAS* |
| WASH. U., SEATTLE | U.C. SAN FRAN. | U.C. SAN FRAN. | U.C. BERKELEY* |
| WASH. U., ST. LOUIS* | WASH. U., SEATTLE | WASH. U., SEATTLE | WASH. U., ST. LOUIS* |
| WISCONSIN* | WASH. U., ST. LOUIS* | WASH. U., ST. LOUIS* | WISCONSIN* |
| YALE* | WISCONSIN* | WISCONSIN* | YALE* |

*Denotes schools leading in both Annual Reviews authorship and in Nobel Prizes.

length articles reporting original research, letters to the editor, professional association news, advance publication of abstracts of conference presentations, staff appointments and obituaries, book reviews and advertising. Pressures since the 1960s, however, have pushed reviews out of many English-language journals. Some of the strongest relate to the lobbying of editors by authors (usually dues-paying, subscribing, and voting society members) to reduce the lag time between acceptance and appearance of manuscripts, and yet accommodate as many papers as possible. These are two mutually conflicting goals: The more papers the editors accept, the greater the backlog. Complicating matters was the fact most review articles take up a great deal of space for both text and lists of references, and that the publication of such a review, however intrinsically valuable, in a narrow political sense, satisfied the demand for space of perhaps one or two authors. The competitors for the same space, by contrast, typically represented several teams of researchers, each with much shorter papers. Many editors and publishers decided that they had to give priority to this larger and more easily accommodated constituency of authors and subscribers. Editors and publishers generally decided to pursue one of three options to create more space at the expense of reviews:

- Editors would simply cut back on the number of reviews. Reviews became an irregularly appearing feature within the journal. This simple adjustment was, ironically, chosen by the fewest journals. However, some of these, such as *Science* and *Nature*, and some important journals in clinical medicine, are weeklies and still provide a rather large number of reviews annually even if each issue no longer has a review.
- Reviews would have to become much shorter, an option that was rarely chosen before the 1970s, because it seemed to both authors and readers so contradictory to the surveying function of the review. Three shifts in attitude made the acceptance of "minireviews" more popular in the seventies. First, minireview authors followed the path of most authors of regular articles, and wrote on much narrower topics than are usually associated with traditional reviews. Second, fewer articles were expected to be cited in a minireview, a savings in article

preparation time, and as a corollary, it was no longer considered arrogant to have the review author's own papers to be predominant among them. Third, *Cell*, the most influential journal of the decade, actively promoted minireviews. (See Figure 6 for a comparison of the reference characteristics of minireviews with traditional reviews.)

- Reviews would have to be eliminated from the regular issues of a journal entirely, and exiled into a special issue solely for reviews, or more commonly, into a freestanding journal for reviews alone. This seemingly radical option was actually the most popular, particularly in larger societies with monthly or semi-monthly journals, that felt that they could not go to a weekly publication schedule. Of course, the exile was not entirely an abandonment by the society. The new journal for reviews would often have a softbound format with obvious links in style and typography to the parent journal. Its frequency would usually be quarterly or bimonthly.

## THE ROLE OF THE FOR-PROFIT SECTOR
## IN PROMOTING SEPARATE SERIALS FOR REVIEWS

Another development that supported the separate publication of journals devoted solely to reviews came from some of the smaller research and professional societies in the U.S. They envied large society perks in publishing but had enough trouble managing their smaller publication programs just as they were. These fledgling societies were happy to let for-profit firms take over much of the marketing, production, and distribution of their publications on a kind of profit-sharing basis. Through these takeovers, those firms multiplied revenues for the smaller societies and for themselves by accelerating a natural tendency for features within the multifeature journals to break off into their own special feature publications. This initially led to separate letters journals, special convention publications, and membership newsletters. That this fragmentation was not protested by the society is explained by a deal with which librarians have become all too familiar. Most of these newly separate journals were initially made available for free or at low cost to society members. Any revenue loss was covered by higher charges

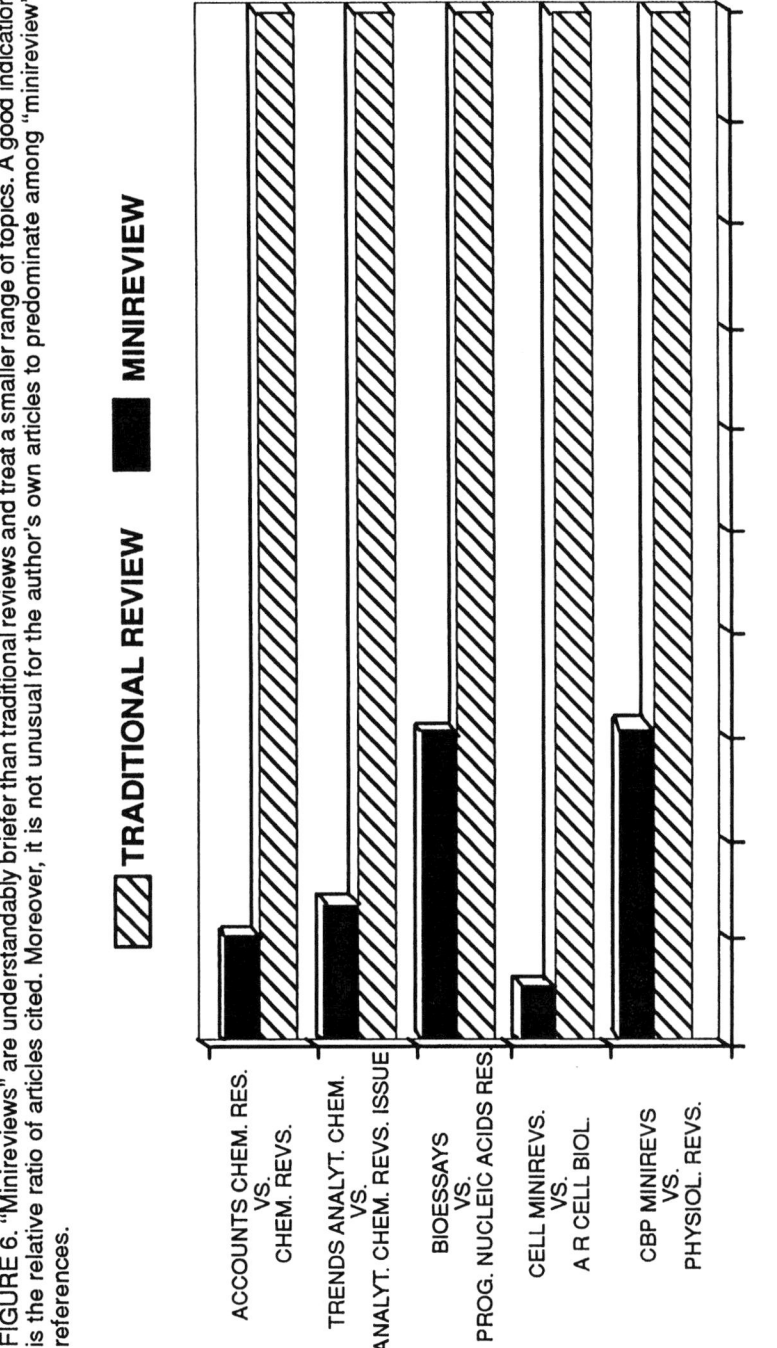

FIGURE 6. "Minireviews" are understandably briefer than traditional reviews and treat a smaller range of topics. A good indication is the relative ratio of articles cited. Moreover, it is not unusual for the author's own articles to predominate among "minireview" references.

15

to third-party subscribers like libraries. This led to the curious fact that with time, many specialty societies no longer sustained at all, an integrated, general purpose journal in which reviews might appear. Since the demand for reviews did not go away–the proliferation of fragmented information sources made reviews even more necessary–separate journals for reviews seemed to be the answer. It no longer mattered as much if the society partner cooperated or not, since the chain reaction both partners had a hand in starting seemed entirely self-sustaining by now. By the 1970s, most separate publications for reviews were being launched by for-profit publishers. Interestingly, most were issued less frequently than those associated with large societies (who still favor quarterlies or bimonthlies), and appeared in a hardbound format (larger societies favor softbounds that strongly resemble their regular journals). These two developments require a look at the European experience for an explanation.

## *HOW THE HARDBOUND FORMAT FOR REVIEWS AND "ANNUAL" PUBLISHING SCHEDULE HAVE EVOLVED*

There have been several Continental European influences on the evolution of hardbound review serials. Antecedents of this genre are actually quite a bit older (generally 19th century) than those dealing with softbound quarterly or bimonthly reviews originating in the English-speaking community (generally the 1930s). A common practice among German, Swiss, Austrian, and Scandinavian societies and universities was the issuance of a hardbound yearbook. Like the general purpose scientific journal, the *Jahrbuch* (Yearbook) or *Jahresbericht* (Annual Report) initially had a number of functions, including data on the state of the discipline in terms of academic programs and publications, theses presented and defended, symposia held, and the inaugural lectures of new professors. But in a reverse of the trends of twentieth century English-language publications, critical surveys of articles published elsewhere became more, rather than less, important with each passing year in "Jahr" publications. Reviews came to dominate this genre. One important irony was that while *Jahresbericht* limited themselves pretty strictly to surveys of literature appearing in the previous year,

*Jahrbücher* stressed lengthy analysis of literature that had appeared in any time span that was pertinent to the subject of the review. The "Jahr" tended to refer more closely to the frequency of publication of the hardbound review volume, rather than to year of appearance of the literature it discussed.

There were a number of reasons why this format and publishing schedule didn't quickly catch on in the U.S.:

- First, most of these publications were in non-English languages, typically in German. While English-speaking graduate students were nominally required to acquire a reading knowledge of German, Americans in particular acquired no taste for freely exercising this skill if it could be avoided. Curiously, the reverse strategy of having American publishers field English-language reviews seemed financially shaky. The number of American schools that might buy them was still small and it was thought that foreign sales of these proposed English-language reviews would be necessary to cover costs. However, such sales were far from certain. The loftier status of foreign language scientific institutions in Europe, and European eagerness to buy and read works published in English, particularly by those rustic Americans, was open to doubt. Continental collections did have the principal English-language journals, but would sophisticated European collectors spend much money on a relatively new genre from such neophytes? Recall that until well after the First World War, most of America's scientific faculties either acquired their Ph.D.'s or did their postdoctoral training in Europe, an acknowledgement of the scientific imbalance of prestige.
- Second, the spheres of influence of existing European "Jahr" publications tended to be limited through old traditions of provincial rivalry. Authorship of reviews was often restricted to the local pool of talent. (Each German university and district society assuming that, of course, its pool of talent was quite sufficient and qualified for the task!) It took a while, even in Europe, for some of the "Jahr" genre to spread beyond their provincial boundaries and for a few of them to become essentially international in reputation and sales.

- Third, most of the actual printers of the works were housed off-campus and were highly independent in some matters of sales and distribution. Unlike the British and American situation, where a certain distinction and hierarchical authority of "publisher" over "printer" was maintained, these German "printers" often effectively became the "publishers" as well. They exercised a stronger control over these yearbooks outside the local community than did the university or society. These printer-publishers did share one conservative judgement with their counterparts in the American publishing community. They did not immediately stress transatlantic distribution, because they saw limited profitability in sales to the U.S., given the costs involved of servicing that initially small demand.

Nonetheless, the "Jahr" genre slowly became more familiar and accumulated respect–in part because the few places that did collect them were so prestigious and trend-setting: Johns Hopkins, the Ivy League, the Big Ten, the rising California universities. These were the places that accumulated the best scientific talent of that day, and as we have seen, that talent regularly studied for a time in Europe and likely brought back a taste for *Jahrbücher* with them. Financial and cultural barriers to acceptance of English-language annuals in Europe lingered into the turn of the century. Then, one segment of the British scientific community, the Chemical Society, scored a smashing success in both the U.S. and European markets through the 1904 inauguration of its *Annual Reports on the Progress of Chemistry*, a kind of *Jahresbericht*.

Americans were particularly happy about the international success of the English language text, but the still small and still shaky American scientific for-profit sector was not ready to jump in. It took an initiative from the nonprofit sector to get serious reviews off the ground in the U.S. Through the foresight of some talented organizers in concert with a quintessentially elite network of early editors and contributors, the *Annual Reviews, Inc.* foundation was established in 1932 in California. Starting initially with the hardbound *Annual Review of Biochemistry* and the *Annual Review of Physiology*, each with a mix of papers that leaned more to a *Jahrbuch* than to a *Jahresbericht* approach, the foundation scored its own breakthrough. Sales worldwide were good enough to help fund a gradual expansion of the series over the years so that by 1991, there were seventeen subject versions. Many are regarded as the leaders in their disciplines, and their formats and publishing schedule are much copied. The J. Murray Luck Award, named after the foundation's guiding light, is given to the best scientific review author in the world annually. Although no preference is given to those who publish in the *Annual Reviews*, it is not surprising, given the reputation of that series for attracting talent, that many award winners have appeared there.

The for-profit segment of the publishing community in both Europe and America responded to the success of this non-profit foundation by fielding their own reviews. Not surprisingly, these were usually issued in roughly annual installments and in hardbound formats. Sales of reviews in German within the U.S. were initially slow, but increased as more of these annuals changed from German language articles to English. The *Fortschritte der* . . . became *Progress in* . . . , and so on. It is important to note that these were not translated journals. At the insistence of their German publishers, most German review authors were now writing directly in English.

Within the U.S., Academic Press (a firm founded by Eastern European immigrants with experience in the scientific literature over there) became the leading commercial publisher of hardbound scientific annuals. Its *Advances in* . . . series is among the most common on library shelves, and has almost as much name-recognition as the *Annual Reviews*. (Alas for Academic and for serials librarians tracking publishers, not all the journals with the *Advances in* . . . title are Academic products, however.)

## THE STYLES OF INDIVIDUAL REVIEW PAPERS

Given the many and sometimes conflicting missions assigned to reviews, it should not be too surprising that a number of different ways of handling the burden are attempted by their authors. Many review authors attempt to undertake only some of these challenges. They place differing emphases on given review article functions to the neglect of others. It is not unusual to mix styles or missions within any given survey. Nonetheless, here are some common approaches to composing a review:

*The Tutorial.* In this style of review, the author begins with fairly basic definitions and attempts to outline what is included or excluded in his or her treatment. The sequence of topics is then treated pedagogically: general concepts are defined and introduced, then particular special cases are handled. While tutorials can contain historical detail, the train of topics is not necessarily in the order that given ideas were announced or proven. (Often isolated special cases of the topic of the tutorial were first discovered before the valid scientific generalization or rule was announced based on accumulating evidence, and this sequence may be more confusing than instructive.) In many respects, however, the tutorial is the most satisfactory style of review for readers new to a field, or for a field that is, itself, fairly new. Its drawback may be the general absence of a feel for ongoing controversies. This type of review is sometimes suitable for a minireview, if the number of topics and references discussed is limited. The tutorial review is very common in mathematics, where such papers are termed "expository." It has more recently become common in other disciplines through Elsevier's *Trends* family of highly readable reviews.

*The Installment Review.* This review works on the assumption that the reader is already fairly conversant with the fundamental literature of the field. It presupposes that the reader may well have read reviews on the topic in the past, but would be appreciative of an update, most often the highlights of the previous year. This style is clearly inherited from the old *Jahresbericht* school, or its latter-day British emulators. Many researchers in specialized fields feel less isolated and less powerless over the flood of the mainstream of information because of their reliance on this style of review with its regular readings of the gauges of current flow of new developments. Chapters in these reviews tend to have the same working titles year-after-year, to facilitate their being scanned by devotees. A fairly neutral, reportorial discussion of developments is expected. These reviews are rarely minireviews, since the broader topical categories in installment plan reviews rarely involve less than a hundred or so references a year.

*The State-of-the-Art Review.* This is the most common type, and like the installment review, it is intended mainly for advanced readers. Most state-of-the-art reviews are not, however, done on a broad specialty within a discipline (the approach of an installment review), but rather on specific topics, ripe for a powerful generalization (full-length, traditional reviews) or demanding of special attention from the rest of the profession (the minireview). There is a length-dependent relationship in the amount of controversy in these reviews. Ironically, the lengthier they are, the more impartial and convincing they seem. To the degree that the traditional review author wishes to make a point, he or she can do so with a more exhaustive examination of all perspectives. There is a subtle "preponderance of evidence approach" in traditional length reviews. This seems to be the style favored by older Americans and most Continental European authors. By contrast, the more controversial state-of-the-art reviews tend to be minireviews, and these are favored by younger American authors. Two assertions often underlie the state-of-the-art minireview. The author explicitly states that his or her work is "hot," and that the particular approach followed in the author's lab is the best available. Opinion is much more frankly stated in these reviews, and examples of supporting and contradicting papers from competing labs are often harshly hashed out in short order. Such reviews usually require some strength of ego on the part of the author, and some tolerance of any author self-indulgence on the part of the reader. The time-frame of references cited is not usually as formally confined as in the installment plan approach, but most of the controversial papers cited involve relatively recent developments on which a consensus has not yet emerged. State-of-the-art minireviews get the reader to the "war-zone" the fastest. Brevity and interest in controversy have allowed for minireviews in some mixed-function journals that would not otherwise have made the space for traditional reviews.

*The Life-and-Times Review.* These are generally of two types. First, there are autobiographical reminiscences that are selectively documented with what the author regards as his or her key papers over time. These references are intermingled with the historical background of the topic under discussion, so that both biographers of science and current practitioners of the scientific specialty of the author can conceivably be served equally. Second, there are life histories of famous scientists, usually accompanied by more or less complete bibliographies, authored by junior colleagues or former students on the occasion of the senior scientist's birthday, retirement, or death. While these can occasionally illuminate a field as much as they do the life of the subject, the biographical portion generally has greater emphasis, particularly when the honoree has had a long career. As a rule, American and British reviews tend to feature more of the first "anecdotal" type, while Continental European publications, particularly from German-speaking countries and the former Soviet Bloc, favor the second, "saga" type. There are also some differences of psychology involved: the Anglo-American, whatever his or her actual deportment, is expected to come across in most reviews as humble, and almost apologetic for taking up this space in a journal, everywhere deflecting praise for any achievements towards colleagues and students. In this tradition, the autobiographer pays tribute to either a kindly senior professor, or to a chance discovery, for having set the writer on a course that proved successful, but which he or she otherwise might not have found for themselves. The goal of western reviews is the humanization of the scientist, and encouragement of neophytes who would follow his or her path.

By contrast, in the Continental European tradition, the subject is generally portrayed as a "wunderkind" from the start, the telling of which usually includes a good deal of ancestral history and childhood documentation. Each report card and examination passed is noted as proof of the almost inexorable advance of the prodigy. Of course, the rich ore of the young scientist is fire-tested and then hammered into steel by working under famously severe taskmasters at the university or research institute of his or her training. Finally, the "call" from the ultimate place of employment and the string of major discoveries is played out. In every reference discussed by the author of the review, it is our hero who broke through the logjam and made it all possible. The goal of Continental reviews is the canonization of the scientist, and the warding off of unworthy amateurs who would enter the domain which he or she carved out masterfully for all time.

# ARE THERE OTHER WAYS IN WHICH SCIENTIFIC PERSPECTIVES CAN BE DRAWN? RECURRING SYMPOSIA AND THEME ISSUE JOURNALS

There are at least two other ways to get the big picture or extensive subject treatments that review journals promise:

- One way, the recurring symposia journal, emphasizes a greater democracy of viewpoints on a subject, often with a livelier presentation.
- A second way, the theme issue journal, emphasizes somewhat greater editorial control than symposia lend themselves to, while still providing a diversity of viewpoints.

Neither of these alternative approaches is as widespread in science as is the review journal. But today, each has given rise to allied literatures that are often treated like review journals by scientific authors, readers, and librarians. Moreover, the costs of these alternative or companion literatures also run into the hundreds of dollars per subscription annually, no small matter in age of library retrenchment. No treatment of review-type literature would be complete without an acknowledgement of their strengths and disadvantages.

# RECURRING SYMPOSIA: WHY THEY SOMETIMES SUCCEED AS INDEPENDENT SERIALS

Symposia feature the in-person presentation of many viewpoints on a topic over a fairly short time, generally at meetings that last from a day to a week. There is a tremendous historical background to the symposium journal. It is arguable that most early scientific journals were initially the transcriptions of meetings of scholars. Consider the large number of society-sponsored journals entitled the *Proceedings*, the *Transactions,* or as the French used to say the *Rendered Accounts.* Of course as scientific disciplines specialized, most of their symposia agendas specialized as well, and most symposia came to deal with a rather narrow range of topics at any one time, not with all the research topics that could conceivably interest the group. Moreover, the growing size of most societies forced a certain restriction on the number of speakers that could be heard in plenary sessions. Not even the Superdome, for example, could seat all the members of the American Chemical Society. Imagine the duration of such a conference if each attendee were granted the right to speak to the general session!

There is today, moreover, some effort at quality control through selectivity in invitations to speak. Keynote speakers are typically chosen for reasons of high professional visibility. Organizers also provide for complementary coverage of topics since speakers can be apportioned different areas of the topic of the symposium. When there is a controversy in a field, it is entirely possible to let each disputant air his or her own presentation. Sometimes, actual debates are held between speakers. Further, it is often easier to get good contributors to a symposium, since each speaker is not personally held accountable for reading and integrating hundreds of prior articles. Speakers just present their own views with only the amount of prior reference that they feel is appropriate. This does not require the speaker to spend so much time away from his or her laboratory. The sense of perspective then, as provided by symposia volumes, is not so much one of many studies compared by a single author over a long time as a comparison of many ongoing studies, initially in the minds of the listening audience, and subsequently in the minds of the symposia volume reader. Finally, some symposia record the from-the-floor remarks and questions following a speech, and any answers the speaker may provide. This can make for livelier reading than is typically found in review articles. With all of these advantages, it may seem surprising that the symposia has not entirely obviated the review journal.

## WHY SYMPOSIA OFTEN FALTER
## AS INDEPENDENT SERIALS

Yet there are only one or two dozen significant symposia series that stand today as successful independent publications in the sciences. For on reflection, there are still many uncertainties in putting together virtually any symposia that do not often occur when producing traditional reviews.

*First*, while symposium participants may be assigned in advance a given topic to cover, there is no way to contain individual remarks once the participants start. A symposium can scarcely tout the prestige of its speakers and then try to refocus their talks in front of a live audience. Consequently, a hoped-for complementarity of presentations at a live symposia can go awry. (Editors of a review journal by contrast, can enforce topical restrictions through discreet private communications that are impractical in a public setting.)

*Second*, the symposium speeches that are the most "listenable" are not often the most readable. Compilers of symposia talks rarely have "courtroom transcribers." They rely on symposium speakers to hand over a "clean" manuscript version of the talk they delivered, ideally making any corrections, substituting illustrations for slides, and omitting parenthetical remarks, and any chatty or comic asides. But speakers at scientific conferences are human, and have a tendency to try to make one version of their talk serve two often contradictory functions: entertainment *vs.* serious analysis. Those speakers who try to compose their oral presentations so as to be easily transferred to print generally end up "reading the pages at their audiences," often resulting in a sleeping audience. Those speakers who give a lively presentation often have a manuscript for later publication that is difficult for readers to follow smoothly. Systematically reworking the speeches, especially when added to the discomforts of traveling to symposia, is often regarded by symposium contributors as a chore almost as burdensome as having to write a single review article once.

*Third*, the democracy implied by the many speakers at a symposium *vs.* the few authors of a review is diminished by the fact that symposia as actual events financially succeed only to the degree that they attract star speakers who will bring in many paying registrants. The lesson of recruiting review authors is not lost on those recruiting symposia speakers: Harvard, Johns Hopkins, Chicago, and the like, tend to dominate the most successful symposia rosters much as they do review journals, since they provide the major source of scientific leaders people are willing to pay to hear. So much for greater democracy! One of the disappointments of both conference organizers and attendees occurs when the invited scientist sends his or her graduate student as a stand-in, without prior notice. The invited but absent scientist argues (somewhat ingenuously) that it is the "content" that matters, not the "mouthpiece." (I think this is the rationale used by Elvis impersonators, by the way.) Disgruntled attendees occasionally vent their anger by sharply grilling the youngster from the floor, an uncomfortable situation for the neophyte in most circumstances, although favored even now as a blood sport by senior scientists in the audience as much as fox hunting was by 19th century British gentry.

By contrast, the highly democratic approach of letting everyone who pays to attend give a talk which is fully reproduced in the symposium volume diminishes the post-symposium sales appeal of the work. Scientific buyers are not eager to spend money on the views of those who are less well-known. A compromise, the provision of briefer abstracts for the talks or "poster sessions" of the "nonstar" presenters, is regarded as a bridesmaid phenomenon. It is like a maid of honor attending too many weddings without ever personally going on a honeymoon: after a while, more depressing for her than not being invited to the wedding at all. She can spend almost as much time and money in preparation for the event as the bride (indeed star speakers, like brides, can expect gifts and expense accounts) but a bridesmaid has a lot less to show for her investment of time and money afterward. Tenure committees and grants reviewers tend to regard as dubious those *vitae* that are full of convention abstracts, but repeatedly lacking in the eventual, full publication of their brief talks or posters. Evaluators begin to suspect that the ideas of the author just don't seem to merit a full printing anywhere.

*Fourth*, symposia series tend to succeed as independently issued serial publications only to the degree that they are promptly issued in print. This is necessary to increase the willingness of good speakers to sign on, and to build the confidence of library subscribers to the proceedings. Those that do the best seem to have substantial outside funding from the very inception of the program –often from scientific supply or pharmaceutical firms–so as to underwrite the expenses of the star speakers, and a permanent site to host the symposium. Corporate seed money and a permanent site help to carry the symposium series along financially until its intrinsic reputation for quality takes over in generating advance sales. Advance orders give publishers money to invest even before the volume is ready, diminishing the financial risks of publishing symposia. Those symposia that are without a good deal of advance, recurring external support can rarely fund themselves out of sales of the volume a year or two after the fact. Who will carry the other costs in the interim?

*Fifth*, in contrast to the experience of review articles being kicked out of multifeature science journals into their own serials, successful symposia tend to get absorbed back into regular journals, losing their independent identity. It is a matter of reducing uncertainties for all concerned. After the incorporation of a symposium issue into a regular journal, seemingly altruistic corporate underwriters of the formerly independent publication of the symposia gladly become frank advertisers. Advertising in unaffiliated symposia journals, in contrast to ads in wider circulation journals, tends to be muted and discreet–often limited to something like the brief opening acknowledgement of sponsorship as seen on nonprofit public television. Multiple, heavy-handed ads in unaffiliated symposia proceedings would convey the impression that the entire conference was somehow "bought" by its usually exclusive sponsor.

With a change to publishing the symposia within a general purpose journal, corporate sponsors actually have more advertising leeway. Since there are usually many different ads in a general purpose journal, their own ads are not open to any charge of censoring or controlling the conference. Corporate sponsors can actually buy a greater amount of space and feature a more obvious sales pitch. Sponsors know that the circulation for the symposium issue (and the exposure of their ads) will be at least as great as the journal's regular circulation. Speakers at such symposia know that the proceedings will be published as part of the regular calendar cycle of the journal and will not have to wait unduly for an independent issuance some time down the road. Harried symposium organizers are also spared the problems of dealing with accountants, printers and distributors that they have individually signed up for each volume. Quite often, they find themselves willing to trade off their publication's independence in return for the reassurance of being associated with a larger professional society or for-profit publisher, and its experienced staff.

*Finally*, it must be acknowledged that symposia serials as a class rarely exceed the impact factors of the review journal competition in their fields. While scientific readers may wish to read many views, they cite a relatively small proportion of them, largely, one suspects, those of the stars. See Figure 7 for a comparison of the impact factors of symposia vs. reviews.

## *THE THEME ISSUE JOURNAL: A SYMPOSIUM WITHOUT AN ACTUAL MEETING*

Those who view the chaos and uncertainty of the symposium with trepidation, but like its multiple viewpoints, have hit upon the theme issue journal. A number of serials which use the word symposium in their titles are, in fact, theme issue journals. In theme issue journals, the editors only figuratively round up the experts on given parts of a topic. (They just write, phone, fax or e-mail them and the separate authors often never meet.) The editors ask the invited authors to write from their own perspectives. Much as is the case with symposium papers, there is no requirement for systematic citation of all previous literature on a subject by each of the theme authors. The correlation of viewpoints is largely left to the reader, although the special editor for each theme issue will sometimes attempt an integrating introduction or afterword. The editor of a theme issue also has the option of asking a contributor to revise his or her paper so as to better fit the announced theme, a rare luxury for "live" symposium organizers.

That theme issue journals are not more common is more of a mystery than the decline of the independently published symposium. But perhaps they have lacked a consistently appearing prototype in the first place. The closest thing to a model for a theme issue journal is the European tradition of the *Festschrift* (loosely translated: "Collection of Commemorative Writings"). *Festschriften* have close affinities in motivation and intent with life-and-times review articles. Generally at the retirement or death of a major scientist, his or her former students contact one another. They form a delegation and go to a publisher, with the idea of a book of essays

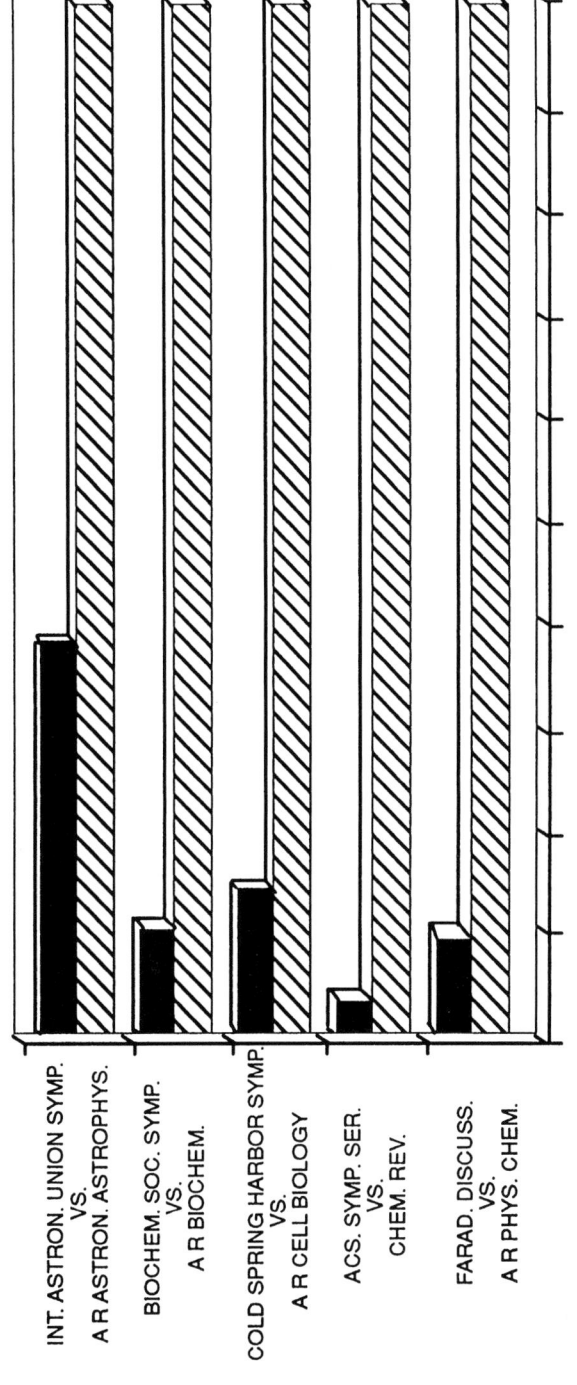

FIGURE 7. While symposia serials have strengths, reviews usually surpass them in impact factor.

TRADITIONAL REVIEW    SYMPOSIA SERIALS

RELATIVE IMPACT FACTOR

INT. ASTRON. UNION SYMP.
VS.
A R ASTRON. ASTROPHYS.

BIOCHEM. SOC. SYMP.
VS.
A R BIOCHEM.

COLD SPRING HARBOR SYMP.
VS.
A R CELL BIOLOGY

ACS. SYMP. SER.
VS.
CHEM. REV.

FARAD. DISCUSS.
VS.
A R PHYS. CHEM.

or a special issue of a journal dealing with the scientific themes pursued by their hero. It is customary for each contributor to acknowledge somewhere in his or her own essay how the early lessons of Herr Doktor Professor made a profound influence on their own current studies. This need not mean that each paper is necessarily backward-looking. Publishers are particularly eager that the appeal of the volume expand beyond those who had a personal affiliation with the honoree, and include material of ongoing research interest.

This need for financial self-support may also play a role in the relative paucity of theme issue journals. There have been few or no *Annual Reviews* type foundations that have consistently underwritten them. Most journals featuring special theme issues have been published by for-profit firms who then sell individual issues to those without a continuing subscription but with an interest in that particular topic. This is a common form of second-wind cost recovery that can reduce the uncertainties of the publisher's investment, if not a librarian's worry about buying the same material twice.

There are also problems of prestige for theme issue journals relative to other types of perspectives serials. Theme issue journals have not been consistently well cited, and certainly fail to pass their review journal competitors in impact factors (see Figure 8). This may have something to do with the fact that theme issue journals, unlike recurring annual symposia and many hardbound reviews, tend to appear more often, most commonly on a quarterly basis. This creates a dilemma of delivering consistently high-interest manuscripts to the readers over the years. With the passing of time, fewer and fewer key themes are still untreated, and, as importantly, the supply of uniformly famous writers is more quickly exhausted. As more and more esoteric topics are treated instead of "hot" topics, fewer devotees of those esoteric topics are to be found among the readers. The less popular themes generate fewer citations to the journal over time. In sum, theme issue journals, while having a number of advantages, do not have the agenda-setting power that review journals command. Each of their more frequent issues is not as likely as an annual review to stir new controversies and redirect careers. Nonetheless, finding a pertinent theme issue for a library customer often repre-

FIGURE 8. While theme issues are attractive, reviews typically have greater impact.

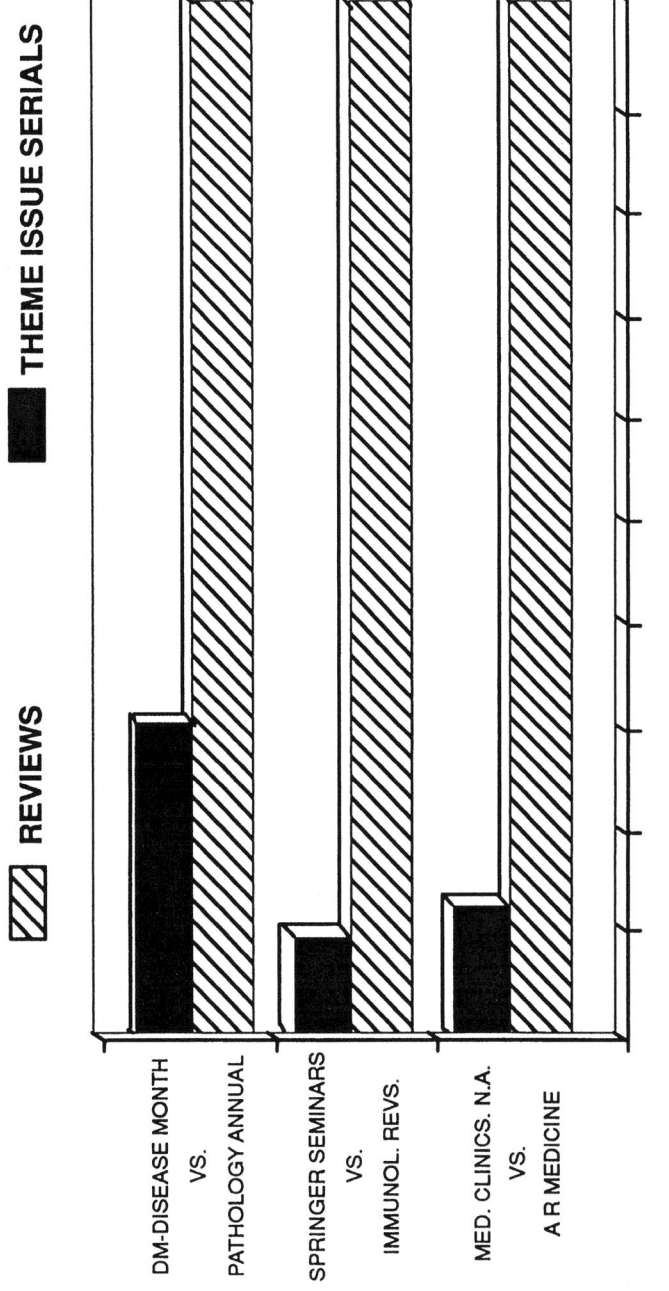

sents a tremendous time-saving for that patron, and this category of materials deserves serious attention.

## THE METHODS SERIES: AN ENCYCLOPEDIA THAT NEVER STOPS BECAUSE THE HUNGER FOR NEW METHODS NEVER GOES AWAY

The 18th and 19th centuries were an era for encyclopedic summations of knowledge. In virtually every major European country, national encyclopedias encompassing "all knowledge" were initiated, sometimes by a single author, but more often under the directorship of a committee of contributors. There were at least two conflicting goals: comprehensiveness and currency. In the overwhelming number of cases, emphasis on the first value sabotaged the second. Many encyclopedia volumes were published out of alphabetical order or other planned sequence. Older volumes were sometimes revised and reprinted before the inaugural appearance of a companion volume even took place. Some encyclopedias were never finished.

The encyclopedic impulse certainly seized the sciences. While a variety of nationalities fielded a number of heavily illustrated, semi-popular natural history encyclopedias, it was the Germans who most forcefully seized upon the systematic, serious disciplinary-specific reference work. The names of Beilstein, Gmelin, and Landolt-Bornstein are historically intertwined with an effort to codify carefully verified facts and procedures in chemistry and physics.

Their original idea was of a *Handbuch*, a guide that literally would fit in one's hand and would serve as a constant companion. But then the handbook physically evolved into an encyclopedia set, and ultimately, became a kind of hyperdetailed indexing-abstracting service of great depth, if of reduced currency. The German-style print *Handbuch*, now sometimes hundreds of volumes per set, is a genre which is in general decline in an age of quick computer retrieval. Costs (in the tens of thousands annually for a subscription) and currency remain tremendous deterrents towards wider subscriptions despite the fact that a number of these *Handbücher* are themselves going on-line in order to remedy their time-lags, if not their costs.

But the need for a recurring review type series focusing on proven methods or on fair comparisons of rival methods has remained strong. Indeed it has greatly increased. Once again, the shrinking of manuscripts in important general purpose research journals has played a key role.

The procedural portions of some manuscripts have shrunk much in the same way as the literature review sections have been reduced within many letters journals. Just as is the case with diminished attention to questions of the intellectual history and motivation underlying experiments, it seems that fewer and fewer practical details enabling a reliable retracing of an experiment are being printed within the articles themselves. Readers are often left to wonder what was the actual technical route to the unfolding of the results being discussed in the article. As more and more scientific frauds come to light, a recounting of accepted protocols is becoming more, rather than less important. The increased propensity "to hide" the exact procedure toward an economically promising new compound or biological agent until it is fully patented, while at the same time announcing its discovery so as to claim credit has added to the concern of many scientists about believability. This may not be helped by having as authors those scientists employed by hi-tech and biotech firms, or scientists having substantial hidden interests through stock holdings in such firms. It is entirely possible that their preliminary pronouncements may be as accurate as those who are financially disinterested in a subject, but suspicions remain. Much of the wealth of America has been based on honest corporate science, but this occurred in an era of much more prompt and complete methodological exposure than seems to be the case today. Today, incomplete disclosure of methodological details is common and there is much cynicism that premature or inaccurate announcements serve more to bolster the price of a company's stock than our understanding as whether or not the pronouncement was accurate. This dearth of attention within the literature to individual procedures and to honest comparisons of the efficiency of competing methods also concerns important but underdiscussed issues such as the infectivity of contaminated materials, the inadvertent release of genetically engineered microorganisms, the potential for carcinogenesis of a chemical or radiation source, and the like. The need for verifiable, safe, and experimentally repeatable guide literature as an antidote is great.

There have been three major responses from publishers to these concerns.

*Modern continuation of the* Handbuch *tradition.* This remains somewhat popular in the physical sciences, the area in which it has its strongest roots. In this approach, the typically hardbound volumes are each assigned a topic, so that volume one might always deal with methods of analysis, volume two might always deal with methods of synthesis, and volume three might deal with methods of safe disposal, and so on. This system works well as long as the individual volumes are revised at about the same time, and each volume stays within its single volume format. Unfortunately, this rarely remains the case. Invariably, progress in volume two is so great that one gets a "volume two part two." This is not to be confused with "volume one, edition two." And volume three is rarely the sum of series one and two, although it is common for the last volume to carry the indexing for all of its numerically preceding companions!

*Occasional publication of extended "consensus" papers within leading specialty journals.* The integration of extensive methods papers with regular papers is most common in clinical medicine. The key to understanding this exception in medicine is that most doctors within a clinical specialty face very similar problems and wish to share information on these common dilemmas so as to reduce uncertainty when dealing with human beings. While consensus papers have many features in common with regular review papers, particularly substantial length and many references, there are at least two notable distinctions. First, in medical consensus papers, there are many authors typically representing several institutions that are geographically remote from one another. The goal is the reinforcement of the success of a given hospital by that of others of good reputation, but of such a distance as to preclude collusion or artifacts peculiar to single locale. Second, there is an intense emphasis on the standardization of procedures followed. Patients are matched as closely as possible. Extraneous factors are systematically ruled out. All the authors follow agreed-upon sampling procedures and statistical tests. The goal of such papers is to provide extreme reliability for the reader facing difficult choices of patient management. Nonetheless, these papers are not popular outside of journals of clinical medicine. This is at least partly because publishing scientists in other fields do not treat the same patients and problems over and over and get much credit for it. The basic scientist's career demands greater attempts at novelty in methods. A successful doctor does not routinely take risks with his patients, whereas a successful scientist might well do so with his samples. Basic scientists further their careers by knowing about standard procedures, and being able to demonstrate that their results are reliable because they used standard procedures. Great credit goes to those who develop methods that remain standard for a long time. But scientists get added credit for discovering improvements to standard procedures that are publishable. In human terms, basic scientists also have somewhat more freedom to make changes in standard procedures when they see fit, because their samples rarely sue them for "going beyond the consensus of opinion." This places "consensus" papers on basic science matters within general purpose journals at a double disadvantage. Like their review paper cousins, they take up a great deal of space, but unlike their clinical cousins, there may not be as much consensus that a given problem deserves this much space. Ten thousand rheumatologists might wish to read a consensus paper on a given medicine for arthritis, because each potential reader treats hundreds of patients with arthritis. But it would be hard to find one thousand chemists who wish to read a long paper on the best way of synthesizing that medicine, because fairly few people in the field are likely to get any credit for duplicating it.

*Publication of separate methods journals.* These differ from the *Handbuch* approach, because most methods journals do not generally attempt to maintain some pre-ordained ratio of topics in each issue or volume. Separate journals for methods concede that improvements in procedures for the different subjects that make up their field may well be uneven over time. Editors of methods journals let the flow of good manuscripts determine what will be published, not some nagging sense that volume two is getting inordinately fatter than volume three, so that volume two's papers ought to be curtailed until volume three catches up. To substitute for the lack of an internal system of indexing as found in *Handbücher*, most methods serials rely on the powerful indexing-abstracting services that cover regular papers in their discipline. In other words, a search for papers on bacterial chromosomes damaged by ultraviolet radiation is likely to bring up papers on a standard method for delivering measured doses of ultraviolet radiation to petri dishes containing bacterial cultures. Separate journals for methods frequently feature review-type articles discussing the relative suitability and accuracy of given approaches. They can serve like a kind of sophisticated *Consumer Reports* for the scientist. Separate journals are the dominant means of communicating methods information in the basic, non-clinical, life sciences. The life sciences have a mix of methods serials: predominantly softbound quarterlies and a few, less frequent hardbounds. A few specialties within chemistry have come to rely on hardbound methods serials that appear annually, but cumulate every five years or decade into something vaguely like *Handbuch*. But the resemblance is superficial. Those chemical works are rarely rearranged and systematized beyond a cumulative index and a handier one-volume binding. Moreover, unlike *Handbücher*, many of their methods "chapters" are covered by the major indexing-abstracting services just as if they were articles in a conventional journal.

*Loose-leaf services covering methods.* The loose leaf format is an attempt to maintain the currency and integrity of a volume dedicated to a single topic by allowing for the substitution of new pages or new chapters for old ones in the same volume. This is an approach that is very common in the literature of law and accounting, where new rulings or regulations modify existing codes all the time. It also serves a small number of scientific disciplines well, when specific, "named" tests are being modified, and only a few pages are being replaced at a time. However, it has not shown itself to be a good method for disseminating the important long survey article comparing the efficacy of rival methods. Even when dealing only with brief additions, the loose-leaf volumes tend to become gigantic over time and suffer from the same out-of-sequence growth that afflicts *Handbücher*. The volume for "Synthesis," for example, becomes three volumes for synthesis. Most of the existing looseleaf services require the librarian to change the indexes to each volume almost as often as he or she inserts new sheets. Few of the respected indexing-abstracting services on which scientists customarily depend cover loose-leaf services. It is likely that on-line retrieval of electronic articles dealing with brief methods reports and modifications will soon give existing loose-leaf methods a run for their money. Longer articles featuring comparative perspectives, however, will likely remain in the print serial domain.

# Advanced Materials, Surface Science, and Failure Analysis

Man began materials science when he started to tailor objects from their natural state to one that suited him better. The phrases "Stone Age," "Bronze Age," and "Iron Age" are expressions of the importance of processed materials in history. Metallurgy is probably the traditional discipline that has given the most impetus to the modern notion of materials science. Alloys have been developed almost continuously for centuries through varying ores, the temperatures of their smelting, and the pressure of their forging. Along with these procedures came the central theme of materials science: changing mixtures and conditions of formulation to get more appropriate properties in a substance. Dissatisfaction with existing materials for some new application, or problems of scarcity and cost, has sustained growth in the field which now has incorporated findings from the formerly isolated fields of textiles, paints, coatings, and solvents, plastics, and ceramics, so that we live today in a world of composite materials.

Materials science has been particularly stimulated through the rise of electronics, computing, and biomedical engineering. Each field presents new demands for customized materials. Many projects also involve thin films: protective coatings for structures, membranes for biotechnology, computer chips for scientific instruments. Many considerations in materials design involve surfaces, boundaries, and interfaces between two differing materials or environments. These can include problems of corrosion, friction, electrical

[Haworth co-indexing entry note]: "Advanced Materials, Surface Science, and Failure Analysis." Stankus, Tony. Co-published simultaneously in *The Serials Librarian* (The Haworth Press, Inc.) Vol. 27, No. 2/3, 1995, pp. 39-44; and: *Special Format Serials and Issues: Annual Review of . . . , Advances in . . . , Symposia on . . . , Methods in . . .* (ed: Tony Stankus) The Haworth Press, Inc., 1995, pp. 39-44. Single or multiple copies of this article are available from The Haworth Document Delivery Service [1-800-342-9678, 9:00 a.m. - 5:00 p.m. (EST)].

*39*

conductance, catalysis. Applied surface science has sprung up to analyze what happens at these junctures and what new technologies might be wrought out of layers only a few atoms thick in many cases.

Finally, there is an old, if somewhat less currently fashionable, tradition within materials science involving failure analysis. This was initially due to the "strength of materials" school in the building sciences and the analysis of stress, vibration, cracks, and metal fatigue in mechanical engineering. For a while, this was the domain of less-schooled technicians, who by contrast with microelectronics materials scientists, dealt primarily with large components that were subjected to fairly simple inspection procedures. This field has become much more instrumentalized and extends analysis of even large-item failures down to the microscopic level, using much more pure science and computer modeling than was formerly the case. In an age of product liability and increased concerns for quality, it has been returning to prominence.

## *REVIEWS IN MATERIALS SCIENCE*

Materials with striking new properties are occasionally covered by reviews in the leading basic science journals, particularly *Science* and *Nature*. Examples include higher temperature superconducting materials and carbon clusters with special structures resembling Buckminister Fuller's geodesic domes, called fullerenes. Journals of applied physics do have materials science reviews from time-to-time. Not surprisingly, these have overwhelmingly stressed solid state materials useful for the semiconductor microelectronics industry.

More materials reviews appear, however, in materials science journals. Reviews within the general purpose journals of materials science fall into two patterns. They are either rare (one or two annually) in such well-established titles as *Materials Research Bulletin* (Pergamon), *Journal of Materials Research* (Materials Research Society), and *Materials Science and Engineering* (Elsevier). Or, they are fairly common (about 6-12 reviews annually) in other standards: the *Journal of Materials Science* (Chapman Hall) and *Materials Chemistry and Physics* (Elsevier). *Materials Characterization* from Elsevier features a "Distinguished Lectures Series" with a strong life-and-times motif. While most of the reviews in any of these materials journals are lengthy and state-of-the-art by intention, there is very frequently a good deal of tutorial detail. This is largely due to the multidisciplinary nature of materials research: the chemists must explain a little chemistry to the metallurgists, the ceramicist outlines a strategy to the polymer person, and so on. This is most clearly found in a regular feature called "The Back to Basics Column" in the journal *Materials Evaluation,* from the American Society for Nondestructive Testing. Tutorial mini-reviews are also a staple of the hottest new journal in the field: *Advanced Materials,* from VCH. Somewhat disappointingly, the new entry from the American Chemical Society, the *Chemistry of Materials,* has not published as many reviews as hoped. Part of the reticence of some of the American materials science titles in carrying frequent reviews is due to the quality and widespread availability of separate vehicles for them.

The leader among serials devoted solely to reviews is clearly the *Annual Review of Material Science* from the not-for-profit Annual Reviews, Inc. It has hit on a winning formula of one introductory essay with a life-and-times format, followed by about a dozen intermediate length state-of-the-art papers. While there is not the annual installment plan of reviews in a fixed array of fields one sees in some British reviews, there has been an attempt in recent years to cover a representative selection from the main conceptual and disciplinary interests within materials science in each volume.

Three competitors stress much lengthier papers: *Critical Reviews of Solid State and Materials Science* from CRC Press, *Materials Science Reports* from Elsevier, and *Progress in Materials Science* from Pergamon. These compete among themselves by price (the CRC price is more modest), and by publishing schedule (while the CRC title is quarterly and each issue has two or more papers, the Elsevier title features one lengthy paper in each of its eight issues). There appears to be some extra emphasis on electronic materials in the CRC title, but such a stress is not unusual in this field. The Pergamon entry probably has the best balance. Priorities in selection here are dependent on whether or not your institution follows the common solid-state bias of the field.

Some of the component and feeder disciplines of materials science have their own review sources. The surface science community is well served by Elsevier's lengthy state-of-the-art *Surface Science Reports,* a largely "dry" vacuum science vehicle, with wet films and certain related emulsions and suspensions particularly emphasized in *Advances in Colloid and Interface Science* from the same publisher. Informal, newsy, minireviews are common in Elsevier's *Advanced Composites Bulletin* and *Advanced Ceramics Report.*

## THEMATIC AND CONFERENCE LITERATURE IN THE MATERIALS AND SURFACE SCIENCE COMMUNITIES

Two series are absolutely key to coverage of conferences on materials science work in the United States. At least twenty times a year, the Materials Research Society publishes its *Symposium Proceedings* in hard-bound, camera-ready format. These are generally the result of a geographically diverse series of "live" seminars organized around a single theme, often a given category of material, type of processing, or testing procedure. This series is very frequently co-sponsored by U.S. federal and military agencies, which may explain its high-quality production and frequency of appearance. Much less frequent, but of similar production quality and format, is a series from the (U.S.) Society for the Advancement of Material and Process Engineering, a group better known by its acronyn: SAMPE. This series is numbered by its year so that one typically has something like the *1994 National SAMPE Technical Conference.* Most of these volumes are also thematic.

The remaining conferences represent either a foreign, or a smaller topical segment of materials science in their coverage. While some American papers do appear in the irregular hardbound and typeset *Current Topics in Materials Science* from Elsevier, it has a Continental European flavor and a hefty per-volume price. There is an even greater European presence and an emphasis on microelectronics materials in the conferences which are covered in *Materials Science and Engineering, A and B.* While this Elsevier title is a general purpose research journal, the conference issues generally run several hundred pages, and account for a good deal of the journal's content. Most, but not all of these special issues are thematic. Likewise, Elsevier's *Applied Surface Science* frequently carries not only conferences but reviews as part of its regular issues.

One group emphasizing a traditional niche within materials, the American Society for Mechanical Engineers, always uses separate publications for its conferences on materials that can stand heat, wear, and vibration. These must be separately ordered through the ASME catalog, where they are accorded an "MD" (Materials Division) serial number. Occasionally one finds symposia in the pages of another journal from a traditional source of large scale materials science, the *Journal of Materials in Civil Engineering* from the American Society for Civil Engineers and the National Research Council of Canada.

## METHODS SERIALS IN MATERIALS SCIENCE

It is almost ludicrous to talk about a distinct methods or procedures journal in materials science, since the entire field is devoted to methods and procedure. It makes more sense to talk of standards literature, and here, series from three publishers are prominent and distinctive.

The first series, the *Treatise on Materials Science and Technology*, consists of dozens of thematic volumes, each containing several exhaustive papers. This series is from Academic Press, a publisher more famous for reviews than for engineering handbooks, and not surprisingly, the individual chapters have a review character, and a uniform, hardbound format.

The second series is actually a pair of publications that work the German *Handbuch* tradition by stressing large compendia of data-filled papers with less text than numerical values and tabular materials. This serial pair consists of the *Special Technical Publications* and *Annual Handbooks* of the American Society for Testing and Materials. While some numbers of these related series are genuine conference proceedings, most are actually periodically revised handbooks for testing given categories of material. Interestingly, a large number of these appear to go quickly out of print, and most seem more readily available as *Books on Demand* from UMI.

Finally, there is a tutorial series from the American Society for Nondestructive Testing. It has the highly novel approach in many of its numbers of using a question and answer format. While this style is probably owing to the trade school tradition in this field, the reference value and practical information on procedures makes this series valuable to many libraries serving large groups of materials scientists. The publisher's catalog, and advertisements in *Materials Characterization* are the best ways to keep up with the current assortment.

# Analytical Chemistry
# in Academic, Clinical, Industrial,
# and Environmental Settings

The need to know what makes up an unknown substance, and to determine the purity of a known substance have long been driving forces in chemistry. Early methods often focused on destructive means: pulverizing by mortar; dissolving in strong acid; melting in crucibles. Determining percentages of components was often impossible because there were few ways to characterize vapors or to reduce residues beyond their slag-like condition.

Major advances occurred in the mid-19th century with the development of hundreds of testing solutions that yielded diagnostic color changes or caused telling precipitations. Inventiveness with scientific glassware, improvements in the sensitivity of scales, and even the standardization of laboratory gas burners all helped increase precision.

Three developments of the twentieth century brought even greater certainty and sensitivity: chromatography, spectroscopy, and computerization.

Chromatography involved better handling of fluids and gases. Both were made fractionable by forcing the gases or fluids to run standardized obstacle courses. These courses were in the forms of specially treated columns or strips, with the specimen often speeded along the course by heat, pressure, or electrical charges. The procedure is called chromatography, from the Greek "chroma" meaning color, because complex biological fluids often separated into com-

[Haworth co-indexing entry note]: "Analytical Chemistry in Academic, Clinical, Industrial, and Environmental Settings." Stankus, Tony. Co-published simultaneously in *The Serials Librarian* (The Haworth Press, Inc.) Vol. 27, No. 2/3, 1995, pp. 45-57; and: *Special Format Serials and Issues: Annual Review of . . . , Advances in . . . , Symposia on . . . , Methods in . . .* (ed: Tony Stankus) The Haworth Press, Inc., 1995, pp. 45-57. Single or multiple copies of this article are available from The Haworth Document Delivery Service [1-800-342-9678, 9:00 a.m. - 5:00 p.m. (EST)].

*45*

ponents distinguished by their colors. Chromatography remains the leading tool of the "separation science" school within analytical chemistry.

The second great advance, spectroscopy, involved a heightened appreciation of the electromagnetic wave-reflecting and wave-absorbing properties of matter. Physicists had long observed that "white" visible light was actually fractionable by a prism into a continuous spectra or rainbow of colored components. Scientists generated much less continuous spectra, with only selected colors showing, by superheating unknown specimens so that they would give off light (similar to the figures of speech "red hot" or "white hot"). They viewed the resulting bands of colors given off through instruments with special prisms or gratings called spectroscopes, and recorded the pattern. Wet, "test-tube" chemistry confirmed the identity of specimens that matched spectroscopic patterns and vice-versa.

Eventually two related conceptual breakthroughs were made in spectroscopy. The first came with the realization that light was but one of many forms of electromagentic wave energy. With the right spectroscopes, wavelengths in portions of the electromagentic spectrum other than those of visible light could also be recorded and used as identification markers. Additionally, bombarding a sample with electromagnetic energy of varying wavelengths (as a substitute in some cases for the superheating of the specimen to obtain visible light) often yielded absorbed or reflected patterns that could be equally informative. Spectroscopy of various wavelengths remains the principal tool of the "signal detection school" within chemical analysis.

The third advance was the rise of computerization. With the microelectronics of computers, instruments could be made that were much faster, more compact, and convenient. Differing chromatographic and spectroscopic procedures could be combined with results compared to patterns stored in the computer's memory. Analytical instruments and analytical scientists became ubiquitous even in smaller colleges, hospitals, food processing industries, and industrial firms.

Three major professional groups within the U.S. attract well over 10,000 members each, representing some of these analysts and their employers. These include the Analytical Division of the American Chemical Society (strong in both academic and industrial membership), the American Association for Clinical Chemistry (overwhelmingly based in pharmaceutical firms, hospitals and for-profit labs that contract with doctors), and the Association of Official Analytical Chemists International (historically, food and agriculture but expanding into personal care products and even biotechnology). The publications of these societies, and several more specialized groups, include several which are very pertinent to our discussion.

## REVIEW SOURCES IN ANALYTICAL CHEMISTRY

Analytical chemistry suffers somewhat from a "familiarity breeds contempt" phenomenon. So much can be done with increasingly common analytical instruments, sometimes down to detection of impurities to parts-per-trillion, or signal sorting despite a veritable forest of spectral peaks in a readout, that most multiscience journals rarely review new developments in analytical chemistry. "Breakthroughs" in sensitivity and speed seem routine. This is sadly true even in many of the standard review sources in general chemistry. Partly as a consequence, chemical analysts have developed an exceptionally robust review literature of their own.

The leading source of reviews is an annual softbound supplement to the leading journal in the field: *Analytical Chemistry*. Each year there are about 25 installment reviews. In even years, they cover given analytical methods or tools like nuclear magnetic resonance spectroscopy and high performance liquid chromatography. In odd years, they cover problem areas of analysis like pharmaceuticals, pollution, the food industry, etc. Every library with any interest in the field at all will want to retain these supplements.

For decades, this eminence has brought few challengers to the fore that attempt to do what *Analytical Chemistry* does in exactly the same way. Two more frequently issued reviews make something of an attempt, varying in that they mix both fundamental, academic papers along with applied, industrial papers in each issue. The length of essays also presents some variation from *Analytical Chemistry*. Somewhat longer state-of-the-art-type papers are found in CRC's *Critical Reviews in Analytical Chemistry*; somewhat shorter surveys are found in Freund's *Reviews of Analytical Chemistry.* While the CRC series has had greater acceptance than has Freund's and attracts more U.S. based authors, both series can be best described as modest successes, needed at the largest institutions but probably not at smaller ones.

By contrast, a tremendously successful entry uses a tutorial and minireview approach, Elsevier's *TrAC: Trends in Analytical Chemistry.* It has outstanding readability, if also a somewhat more heavily European and academic approach to topics and authors than does its competition. It is the clear second choice for all analytical collections, after the special issues of *Analytical Chemistry.* A U.S. trade journal of long standing, *American Laboratory*, from International Scientific Communications, seems to be evolving in a way similar to *TrAC*, although the papers are still longer, less immediately accessible to beginners, and definitely more industrial. It is nonetheless becoming an improved title for smaller academic libraries. It retains a substantial advantage over the pricey Elsevier series, but ranks in necessity only with the *Critical Reviews* and *Reviews of Analytical Chemistry.*

Certain review sources are specialized by instrumental class, and taking them is dependent at least partly on local investment in the featured technology. The leader in chromatography is *LC-GC* from Aster Publishing, a mixed trade-journal/tutorial-journal which covers both liquid and gas chromatography. It has both an American and an International Edition. Lengthier state-of-the-art surveys are found in the irregular series from Dekker, *Advances in Chromatography*, and larger university or industrial collections will also take it. An even more specialized title, but one with wide appeal owing to the great successes the high-pressure, high-performance technique has enjoyed over the last two decades, is *HPLC: Advances and Perspectives* from Academic Press. Pharmaceutical labs, in particular, will regard it as essential.

*Spectrochimica Acta Reviews* from Pergamon/Elsevier dominates most areas of chemical spectroscopy. Few review journals that specialize by given spectroscopic wavelength, techniques or applications have sprung up to challenge it. It certainly remains the first choice for academic collections. *Applied Spectroscopy Reviews* from Dekker is its closest competitor. Its comparative strength is a somewhat greater focus on "real-life" problem-solving reviews. It is recommended in industrial and pharmaceutical collections as an adjunct to the Pergamon/Elsevier title.

## SHARED INTERESTS IN SPECTROSCOPY AMONG ANALYTICAL AND PHYSICAL SPECIALISTS

The selection of serials that are more specialized by differing types of spectroscopy requires somewhat greater sophistication in judgement. It should be noted, for example, that many nuclear magnetic resonance journals in recent years have turned from analytical applications to problems of biomedical imaging, and are not as appropriate as they once were for straightforward chemistry collections. However, sharing an interest with another discipline is not anathema for analytical collection policy. Some spectroscopy journals are dominated by the interests of atomic, molecular or optical physicists and physical chemists, and yet remain of high value to analytical scientists. This is owing to a certain complementarity of interests. The physical scientists are interested in the transitions of physical states of known atoms and molecules, often monitoring them by shifts in wave behavior. Analytical scientists look at the wavelengths or other spectroscopic properties recorded by the physical scientists, as signals that can be diagnostic in the many practical situations of analysts when they don't know the identity of the atoms and molecules in the first place.

Fortunately, the review literature of physical chemistry is compact, and relatively inexpensive. Analytical scientists can stay on top of the big issues through subscriptions to the *Annual Review of Physical Chemistry*, from the non-profit Annual Reviews, Inc. (medium length state-of-the-art papers) and the Royal Society of Chemistry's *Annual Reports on the Progress of Chemistry. Section C. Physical Chemistry* (installment reviews). Both are good, with the former essential in any chemistry library, and the latter still affordable even in moderate sized collections.

Three major reviews cover nuclear magnetic resonance. These are Academic's hardbound *Annual Reports on NMR Spectroscopy*, *Progress in Nuclear Magnetic Resonance Spectroscopy* from Pergamon/Elsevier (a bimonthly softbound), and *Nuclear Magnetic Res-*

*onance,* a somewhat irregular hardbound from the Royal Society of Chemistry, part of a particularly distinguished series which will be discussed shortly. The first two feature lengthy state-of-the-art papers; the third, installment reviews.

The Royal Society of Chemistry is particularly strong in its family of irregular hardbound, installment review sources: the *Specialist Periodical Reports,* of which the aformentioned *Nuclear Magnetic Resonance* is a fine representative. Among the other titles pertinent to our analytical purposes are the *Electron Spin Resonance* and *Spectroscopic Properties of Inorganic and Organometallic Compounds.* Selection is, once again, dependent on local investments in instrumentation and types of chemical species analyzed.

## REVIEWS IN ANALYTICAL JOURNALS
## THAT FEATURE MANY TYPES OF ARTICLES

Most of the competitors of *Analytical Chemistry* feature occasional reviews alongside their regular content. General analytical journals with a significant number of reviews annually include *Analytica Chimica Acta* from Elsevier, and *Analusis,* from the Societe Francaise de Chimique. Both tend to use the state-of-the-art approach. *Microchemical Journal* from Academic, by contrast, favors tutorials. Life-and-times reviews are frequently found in *Clinical Chemistry,* the flagship of the American Association for Clinical Chemistry.

On the whole, chromatography journals feature more reviews than do those of spectroscopy. *HRC: The Journal of High Resolution Chromatography* from Huthig, works the state-of-the art approach, while the *Journal of Chromatography* from Elsevier, features many installment reviews in recurring topics, a factor that is often overlooked by those put off by its considerable price. The *Journal of Chromatography* also features annually a generous, classified bibliography based on analytical methods and areas of applications, that can prove extremely valuable.

*Applied Spectroscopy,* from the Society for Applied Spectroscopy, is somewhat unusual among analytical journals in carrying many life-and-times minireviews of award winning spectroscopists.

## SYMPOSIA AND THEME ISSUE SOURCES IN ANALYTICAL CHEMISTRY

American analytical chemists seem to meet more often than many other chemists in the U.S. Part of this is due to the fact that makers of specialty instruments and reagents often underwrite the costs of some rather grand expositions in order to display their wares before these potential buyers. Summary coverage of the annual "Pittsburgh" conference can be found in many of the newsmagazines of chemistry and chemical engineering, particularly in *Chemical and Engineering News*. (It should be noted that these "Pittcon's" are no longer exclusively held in Pittsburgh.) However, relatively few talks are printed in full, and these often appear in several different analytical journals, particularly those of given methods. The next largest convocations in analytical work are typically sponsored by medically or pharmaceutically oriented workers. Their plenary speeches are generally featured in *Clinical Chemistry*. This journal has actually expanded both the number of talks and the number of meetings it has included in recent years, covering major events such as the National Academy of Clinical Chemistry Symposium, the Clinical Chemistry Forum, the Beckmann Institutes, and the Oak Ridge and San Diego meetings.

The international conference literature scene is also complex, and conference talks–in full or summarized–appear in a wide variety of journals. The British frequently hold conferences, but rarely publish the full text of them. *Analytical Proceedings,* from the Royal Society of Chemistry, provides more summary coverage on U.K. meetings than any other source, although the journal is not exclusively devoted to it, and includes many short papers and news items. The best Continental European conferences seem to appear in *Talanta*, a Pergamon/Elsevier journal. *Talanta* also features many theme issues along the lines of "Analytical Chemistry in Russia," "Recent Advances in the People's Republic of China," etc. A close second in Continental importance are collections appearing in *Fresenius' Journal of Analytical Chemistry*, from VCH, the publishing arm of the German Chemical Society. Interestingly, Fresenius has begun to follow the American practice of providing the full text only for major talks, with a few pages each, at most, for the generally more numerous "poster sessions."

Conference coverage devoted to specific methods of analysis is more occasionally found in journals of spectroscopy and chromatography. *Spectrochimica Acta Reviews* sometimes departs from its review format for symposia papers; the *Journal of Chromatography* can easily find space for several meetings annually in its over 10,000 pages annually.

## METHODS SERIALS IN ANALYTICAL CHEMISTRY

It is awkward to speak of a separate "methods" literature within analytical chemistry. Virtually all analytical journals are overwhelmingly concerned with methods! For chromatographers and spectroscopists, the methodological journey is often more important than the particular analytical question that began their investigation. It is therefore not particularly helpful for discriminating selection to list all the journals of analytical chemistry with an emphasis on methods. The discussion that follows deals largely with two categories of materials. First, there are certain reference sources, issued on a recurring basis, that are of general utility to analysts. Second, we discuss journals dealing with more specialized analytical techniques or instrumentation not mentioned earlier.

The analysis of many everyday materials, particularly in the agricultural, food and other products areas, is covered by the *AOAC International Official Methods of Analysis* guide. Issued every five years, it has annual updates between revised compilations. A similar irregular hardbound, *Standard Methods for the Examination of Water and Wastewater,* from a consortium of societies headed by the American Public Health Association, is an extremely worthwhile companion. Both series are strongly recommended for virtually every analytical collection that deals with real-life applications.

Both industrial and academic collections will also need *Reagent Chemicals* from the American Chemical Society. It contains the standards of purity of many common laboratory chemicals.

Clinical chemists, particularly those assisting pathologists, pharmacologists, and toxicologists with detection of traces of compounds in biological fluids or specimens, will find the *Sigma-Aldrich Handbook of Stains, Dyes, and Indicators* a necessary tool.

The fact that it is a faintly disguised sales catalog for the two related firms does not detract from its high utility.

Two additional hardbound series of great lineage strongly commend themselves to large academic collections. *Techniques of Chemistry* and *Physical Methods of Chemistry*, and their antecedents, have evolved over thirty years into hardbound, theme volumes devoted to given methods, categories of instrument, or classic areas of chemical properties investigation. These series from Wiley are revised irregularly with many volumes having been updated and rewritten a number of times. Eventually, so many piecemeal revisions have accrued that the whole set undergoes a coordinated overhaul and a new edition is announced. The editors attempt to preserve the topical-volume-to-topical-volume lineage as much as possible, while adding new volume numbers for new topics. As the title suggests, physical chemists will also share an interest in at least the latter of these two series.

Larger analytical collections may also wish to subscribe to certain regular serials devoted to new developments in instrumentation or the further automation and integration of separate analytical technologies. Two series come from the physics community and have longevity on their side. These are the *Review of Scientific Instruments* from the American Institute of Physics, and *Measurement Science and Technology* from the (British) Institute of Physics. Since many instruments come to analytical chemistry from physics usages, these have some value. Perhaps greater immediacy, however, is available in three chemically oriented journals. These are *Analytical Instrumentation* from Dekker, *Chemometrics and Intelligent Laboratory Systems* from Elsevier, and the *Journal of Chemometrics* from the British wing of Wiley. The first title has a somewhat greater focus on American authors. However, the second title probably has taken the lead in worldwide practices and developments and might be preferred when only one can be afforded. All of these titles, physical or chemical in origin, ought to be taken in any collection serving the scientific instrument industry.

Electrochemistry is the most common of the analytical approaches not yet mentioned, and is not a particularly expensive technology. It has a very long history in connection with the physical chemistry of solutions, particularly the bulk coating of metals.

But until the advent of microelectronics industry, it was in an eclipse of academic interest and corporate investment. Now, electrochemical literature is of particular importance in the engineering of thin surfaces and the construction of diagnostic electrodes and probes. Over the years, *Electrochimica Acta* from Pergamon/Elsevier, and the *Electrochemical Society Journal* have become the least analytically oriented, and a relatively new title, *Electroanalysis* from VCH, the most focused on analytical signal detection. The traditional leader, the *Journal of Electroanalytical Chemistry* from Elsevier, is somewhere in between topically, but its massive volume puts it in the top of the cost column. Smaller collections, particularly in academia, will make do with *Electroanalysis*. A relatively new title, the *Journal of Trace and Microprobe Analysis* from Dekker, is of particular interest to makers and users of compact or portable electrochemical testers.

Mass spectrometry is another analytical approach to be mentioned. Spectrometry is a separation science approach to analysis that nonetheless shares certain aspects of spectroscopy, hence its similar name. Formerly an expensive and bulky technology, and used largely in the bigger universities and corporations, it is now seeing increasing use in medical and environmental settings. Two publishers, Elsevier and Wiley, have competing families of journals. Historically, Elsevier had the journal of record, the *International Journal of Mass Spectrometry and Ion Processes*, a title whose annual space requirements seemed to equal those of the machine it covered! In recent years, partly in response to complaints of cost and space, Elsevier has also issued the *Journal of the American Society for Mass Spectrometry* at about 10% of the cost. The newer title has become the leader in U.S. circulation, and is recommended for even the smallest facility supporting mass spectrometry.

Wiley has four pertinent titles, divided along both functional and subject specialty lines. Wiley's *Mass Spectrometry Reviews* is the leader in the field. Its state-of-the-art surveys are more cited than the installment reviews of the Royal Society of Chemistry's *Mass Spectrometry*, although both sources are quite worthwhile. Likewise, a quickly rising star has been Wiley's *Rapid Communications in Mass Spectrometry*. It has a general applicability and popularity akin to Elsevier's "American" entry, and is a suitable companion. Wiley's edge for some segments of the "mass spec" community lies in its two, longstanding subspecialty journals. These are *OMS: Organic Mass Spectometry,* which is generally focused on industrial hydrocarbons and polymers, and a clinical and environmental title, *Biological Mass Spectrometry.* In either specialized situation, one of these may substitute for a more generalized title.

An older analytical technology related to mass spectrometry is atomic spectrometry. Despite substantial economic advantages over its relation, both atomic emission and absorption analyses are still most commonly conducted at larger academic and engineering schools and major industrial firms. Its supporting literature is very compact, consisting principally of two journals: the *Journal of Analytical Atomic Spectrometry* from the Royal Society of Chemistry, arguably the academic leader, and *Atomic Spectrometry,* the trade magazine from Perkin Elmer, a leading instrument maker. Both journals provide substantial methodological support and can be afforded at most places where atomic spectrometry is important.

The most important variant within chromatography is the use of thin layer or electrophoretic technology. Here the progress of the "unknowns" across thin slabs of gel or specially treated papers is generally accelerated by an attracting electric current. While the technique has many academic, industrial and agricultural uses, its principal arena is in the biomedical/biotechnological arena. Its sensitivity for the sorting out of various protein or nucleic acid fragments is well developed, and inexpensive kits, or modules insertable into automated lab arrays, are very common in hospital diagnostic labs. (Millions of AIDS tests, for example, use this technology.) While the various journals of clinical chemistry and pathology cover practical methodological examples as a matter of course, more fundamental improvements and highly novel applications appear in analytical journals that appeal to more than just the hospital crowd. The *Journal of Chromatography* and its available subsection, the *Journal of Chromatography–Biomedical Applications* certainly cover the field extensively, and sole reliance on these is feasible in areas where there is already a commitment to their substantial cost. In places where neither of these warhorses is taken, nor the practice of thin-layer work particularly emphasized, one to three specialty titles ought to be considered. *Electrophoresis* from VCH has the widest range of topics, and is senior in standing. Huthig's *Journal of Planar Chromatography–Modern TLC* is a derivative of its longstanding journal *HRC*, and is a good second choice. The newest entry, *Applied and Theoretical Electrophoresis* from Macmillan, shows promise, particularly in light of Macmillan's increasing moves into biotechnology journals.

## THE SPECIAL CASE OF ENVIRONMENTAL POLLUTION MONITORING AND MANAGEMENT

The greatest growth in applied analytical literature over the last 30 years has been in the detection of toxic substances in the environment. The sorting out of the appropriate review, meetings, and methods literature is complicated by a sorting out of the field into increasingly segregated divisions: the field biology of ecology vs. the analytical chemistry of pollution. Few ecology journals, for example, are today focused on detecting contaminants. Academic ecologists have come to concern themselves primarily with inter-species competition, plant and animal interactions, reproductive strategies, the cycling of nutrients in ecosystems, resource depletion, etc. This brief section, by contrast, focuses on literature supporting the use of scientific instruments to detect and sometimes filter out or neutralize pollutants. Virtually all the literature is heavily methodological. Some of the journals from the sanitary engineering constituencies deal with continuous sampling or bulk process treatments of effluents. Several of these titles feature special meetings' issues and buyer's guides.

The leading source devoted solely to reviews is CRC's *Critical Reviews in Environmental Science and Technology*. A softbound quarterly, it is substantially more chemical and toxicological than the *Annual Review of Ecology and Systematics*, the leading review for field biologists. Arguably the most important reviews in a multi-feature journal within the field are in *Environmental Science and Technology*. This American Chemical Society journal is the premier outlet globally, although there are important contributions from other professional groups within the U.S. and strong journals from for-profit publishers here and abroad.

Among the U.S. societies that have long been concerned with environmental quality monitoring are the the Water Environment Federation (*Water Environment and Technology* and *Water Environment Research*) and the Air and Waste Management Association (*Air and Waste Management Association Journal*). U.S. for-profit titles of particular note include Wiley's *Environmental Toxicology and Water Quality.*

British and European titles tend to be issued almost exclusively by for-profit publishers. Pergamon's *Chemosphere* is arguably the best known journal from outside the U.S., although Kluwer's *Water, Air, and Soil Pollution* is rising in importance. In recent years both competitors have introduced sister journals alongside their pioneering efforts: Pergamon has established *Environmental Toxicology and Chemistry*; Kluwer is now fielding *Environmental Monitoring and Assessment.* It is likely that both titles will achieve the prominence of their forebears.

Springer has a longstanding pair of journals that are somewhat more biological than the remainder in this group, but still worthwhile in comprehensive collections. These are the *Bulletin of Environmental Contamination and Toxicology* and the *Archives of Environmental Toxicology.* Elsevier has another somewhat biological entry in *Environmental Pollution.* Interestingly, this last title used to have a separately issued, chemically-oriented title that has been merged back into its parent journal. The case for inclusion of these "biological" titles is made stronger by joint use of the library by wildlife pathologists or public health authorities who monitor specimens as "bio-indicators" of prospective damage to humans.

# Astronomy, Astrophysics, and Space Sciences

Galaxies, gravitational theories, and creation-of-the-universe scenarios dominate most journals of astronomy and astrophysics. Interest in the moon, planets, comets, and asteroids continues, but the bulk of publishing support for these non-stellar objects now seems to come from the geophysical community. This has been a relatively recent phenomenon, and an understanding of its history is important for collection management.

A great deal of the expansion of the geophysical community into space has been commercially, militarily and politically funded, with purely scientific reasons often secondary. Moreover, much of what we have sent up into space was eventually designed to turn around and tell us something about earth, or to improve an earthly situation. Consider the following examples. The limited range of earthbound broadcast signals and problems with atmospheric interference made commercial communications satellites highly desirable. Weather satellites made commuting, shipping, and farming less prone to sudden insurance losses through total unpreparedness. Military support for spies in the sky wasn't based on threats of UFOs from another galaxy, but on missile launches from one part of the earth to another. Public funding for launch vehicles and manned space flights has continued long after we won the political prestige prize by beating the Russians to the moon because environmental change monitoring has been offered as an earth-oriented justification that even fiscal conservatives and antimilitary liberals could support.

[Haworth co-indexing entry note]: "Astronomy, Astrophysics, and Space Sciences." Stankus, Tony. Co-published simultaneously in *The Serials Librarian* (The Haworth Press, Inc.) Vol. 27, No. 2/3, 1995, pp. 59-65; and: *Special Format Serials and Issues: Annual Review of . . . , Advances in . . . , Symposia on . . . , Methods in . . .* (ed: Tony Stankus) The Haworth Press, Inc., 1995, pp. 59-65. Single or multiple copies of this article are available from The Haworth Document Delivery Service [1-800-342-9678, 9:00 a.m. - 5:00 p.m. (EST)].

*59*

The geophysical community that benefited from this buildup had itself built up a tremendous backlog of manuscripts, and understandably wanted to have journals under their control in which these papers could be placed. Librarians should therefore be aware of a nuance when encountering the phrase "space science" as a part of a title in this chapter or in their libraries. Two words–"near" and "deep"–are generally absent from these titles but strongly implied. Understanding this can help clarify distinctions of journal emphasis. Many seemingly generic "space science" journals actually tend to emphasize "near" space objects: planets, their atmospheres, and the interactions of these with the solar wind and with cosmic radiation. Astronomy and astrophysics journals, by contrast, deal largely with "deep space" objects, generally beyond our own solar system.

There is also a difference between "near space" and "deep space" journals based on active versus passive energetics. While some deep space objects are seemingly inert clouds of dust and passively ionized gases–and other objects like neutron stars and black holes have strange gravitational energy situations–most objects of astrophysical interest are actively thermonuclearly energetic. They radiate energy drawn from their own internal fusion. While planets may have molten interiors and even violent surface activity, most of their energy is passively received from a stellar source. Our own sun can be justifiably claimed as a journal topic by both sides. Energetic processes within the sun are largely the domain of astrophysicists. Solar emissions that go beyond the corona to reach the planets are claimed by atmospheric geoscientists. (Particle physicists claim any solar neutrinos that reach their underground detectors.)

While the exciting expansion of the near space sciences has been the biggest story of the the 1950s through the 1980s, the deep space sciences are undergoing a 1990s revival of their own. Despite the initial problems of the orbiting Hubble telescope, new ground-based composite telescopes and computer-guided telescope arrays intended for deep space work have been funded in the past decade and several are successfully coming online even now. The images that they have been bringing in, often further enhanced by computer, have stimulated more academic papers, popular news items, and enthusiasm than have been seen in other recent decades.

# REVIEWS OF ASTRONOMY, ASTROPHYSICS, AND SPACE SCIENCES IN MORE GENERAL SOURCES

Astronomy and astrophysics are very well served by review papers, both from the larger scientific community and from within their own specialty ranks. While it takes a fairly unusual event like Supernova 1987a, or the finding of a new deep-space object to generate a flurry of reviews, important astronomical and astrophysical reviews are not uncommon (4-6 annually) in the British journal *Nature*, and somewhat common (1-3) in *Science*, from the American Association for the Advancement of Science. The general physics community will also publish astronomical and astrophysical reviews in important outlets such as the *Review of Modern Physics* from the American Institute of Physics, and *Reports on the Progress of Physics* from the (British) Institute of Physics, and Elsevier's *Physics Reports*. These are first priority choices, and are likely to be in most physical sciences collections already. *Rivista del Nuovo Cimento* from the Italian Physical Society has a penchant for both gravitational and particle physics papers that are of interest to astrophysics.

# REVIEWS IN GENERAL JOURNALS OF ASTRONOMY, ASTROPHYSICS, AND SPACE SCIENCES

Reviews are occasional items in several of the principal outlets for original research in astronomy and astrophysics. *Astronomical Journal*, an American Institute of Physics title, imbeds them among the regular papers, as does the *Publications of the Astronomical Society of the Pacific*. Both of these favor state-of-the-art reviews. Historical reviews, especially a kind of life-and-times minireview, can be found in the extended obituaries seen in the *Quarterly Journal of the Royal Astronomical Society*, a title handled by Blackwell. This British journal also features a kind of annual installment review detailing progress in British university programs, material that is of high interest internationally given the standing of British work in the field.

## SOURCES SPECIFICALLY DEVOTED
## TO ASTRONOMICAL, ASTROPHYSICAL,
## AND SPACE SCIENCE REVIEWS

Most astronomical and astrophysical reviews, however, appear in an assortment of publications designed principally for that mission. As is frequently the case, the not-for-profit Annual Reviews, Inc. fields the leading overrview title in the discipline: the *Annual Reviews of Astronomy and Astrophysics*. This inexpensive hardbound is absolutely essential for any collection with even a marginal interest in the field. It follows its usual format of a lead-off life-and-times review that is generally autobiographical and follows with a dozen or so intemediate-length state-of-the-art surveys.

Until recently, the survey of second choice has automatically been Kluwer's *Space Science Reviews*. Kluwer has an immense presence in astronomical and astrophysical literature, and this Kluwer entry has competed successfully by featuring some of the longest state-of-the-art reviews in the field, in a somewhat expensive, but generally welcome quarterly softbound format. But Springer, who scooped Kluwer's predecessors twenty years ago by fusing together *Astronomy and Astrophysics,* is once again challenging with *Astronomy and Astrophysics Review.* The Kluwer and Springer entries are now approximately equal in quality and in selection priority. Together with the *Annual Review*, these three are key to any program that offers regular instruction in the space sciences. Nonetheless, two other reviews are to be taken seriously in any collection with graduate instruction.

The second tier of reviews includes a Harwood title: *Comments on Astrophysics,* and a title from Pergamon: *Vistas in Astronomy.* Each has its appeal. *Comments* features a format that combines both a minireview and a thematic issue function. Many of the papers are frank and informal and there are even tutorial items, such as might be seen in workshops for those new to the theme of the issue. *Comments* has seen a number of scope adjustments, and in its current incarnation, takes papers on near-space and planetary topics as well as on stellar and deep-space topics. *Vistas in Astronomy,* by contrast, remains stable in topical scope, but charmingly idiosyncratic in format. Papers range freely from historical and life-and-times themes to more conventional state-of-the art-surveys. In more recent years, subscribers have had the option of taking quarterly softbounds or a hardbound annual compilation.

## THEME ISSUES AND SYMPOSIA IN ASTRONOMY, ASTROPHYSICS, AND SPACE SCIENCES

The leader in worldwide symposia publishing for this discipline is unsurprisingly Kluwer. They are the principal foreign publishers of the numerous and essential *International Astronomical Union: Proceedings of Symposia*, generally cited in the literature as the *IAU Symposia Proceedings*. Kluwer also features symposia and theme issues in its *Earth, Moon, and Planets*; *Solar Physics*; and *Astrophysics and Space Science.* (Some of these are papers extracted from larger *IAU Symposia*.) Kluwer also publishes many of the *NATO Advanced Study Institutes Series.* While most of these deal with European conferences on advanced solid-state technology, or with particle physics, a small number of important astrophysical conferences are issued as *Series B* or *Series C* volumes. Kluwer's only serious competition for European conference work comes from occasional theme or conference issues in *Astronomische Nachrichten*, a former East German vehicle from Akademie Verlag, which generally featured Eastern European work, and from a pair of British-based outlets. The UK outlets have been the semi-popular *Observatory*, which features meeting notes, and the occasional theme issues in *Planetary and Space Science*, from Pergamon.

U.S. conference publishing has been dominated by a regularly issued journal and by two important irregular series. The leader among the regular journals is the *Bulletin of the American Astronomical Society*, which emphasizes meetings abstracts. In the irregular category are publications of the Astronomical Society of the Pacific and from NASA, which generally include full text. The *Conference Series of the Astronomical Society of the Pacific* is a leader in deeper space objects, and has made substantial inroads of late into Kluwer's share of *IAU Symposia Proceedings*. The ASP offers substantial price advantages, good quality, and most small-to-medium libraries will be able to collect their titles. Through its irregular *NASA–SP* series, however, the National Aeronautics and

Space Administration is far and away the leader in publishing formal conference and informal workshop papers done by Americans, including many with near space topics. These softbound, often camera-ready-copy "special publications" now number over a thousand and are required in any large, graduate institution in the field. Historically they have been available at little or no cost through NASA, making their collection well worth their considerable bulk. Cutbacks in federal subsidies may make judicious selection and retention wiser for crowded libraries, as opposed to having the library sign on as a depository for the complete run.

## *METHODS INFORMATION*

Methods papers appear occasionally and without any special designation in leading general purpose titles such as the *Astrophysical Journal*, and the *Monthly Notices of the Royal Astronomical Society*. By contrast, methods papers are flagged in other reputable competitors. For example, the *Publications of the Astronomical Society of the Pacific* has a section on "Instruments and Data Analysis," while *Astronomy and Astrophysics* runs a feature on "Instruments, Data Processing, and Computational Methods." Probably the only journal devoted primarily to these issues is Kluwer's *Experimental Astronomy.* It is recommended for every working observatory and astrophysical lab.

To a great degree, the astronomical observatory is dependent on engineering specialists, a situation not unlike that seen in large experimental particle physics installations. The most pertinent group of technical consultants is the Society of Photo-Optical Instrumentation Engineers. Their journal, generally cited as the *SPIE Proceedings,* is really a collection of hundreds of individually published workshop and/or tutorial papers. While a great many of these deal with more practical, industrial topics, a fair number each year are of interest for astronomical instrumentation. Many observatories retain these selectively.

The geophysical contingent within space science will need occasional access to the publication of another technical group: the Institute of Electrical and Electronics Engineers. The *IEEE Transactions on Nuclear Science* contains papers and conferences on radiation detectors, both ground and satellite based. The American Geophysical Union covers a great deal of information on the detection and managment of transmission disturbances within the atmosphere, including solar burst activity, in its own venerable *Radio Science.*

Finally, some contact of both the geophysical and astrophysical community ought to be maintained to the launch vehicle and satellite engineering community. Technical papers from these engineers tend to give the more basic scientists served in this chapter a sense of the limits and reliability of current machinery. A reasonable collection would include the *Journal of Spacecraft and Rockets*, the most scholarly of several worthwhile publications from the American Institute of Aeronautics and Astronautics, and the *ESA Journal* from the European Space Agency.

# Biochemistry and Molecular Biology

Biochemistry is the study of the more complex molecules that make up cells, or the aggregates of specialized cells we call tissue, which play a significant role in the maintenance of those cells and tissues. Ordinarily, water, oxygen, carbon dioxide, and common salts are not considered to be biochemicals. (Metal ions and metal-containing compounds are certainly important, but are treated in this book as "bioinorganics" under inorganic chemistry.) Literally tens of thousands of carbohydrates, lipids, proteins and nucleic acids, however, do fit the definition.

Each of these four major categories of biochemicals has a primary job in the cell and one or more secondary tasks. The job descriptions vary somewhat among microorganisms, plant and animal cells. On the whole carbohydrates serve a role as energy sources, with extra duties as cell wall material in most plants. Lipids are doubly concentrated as energy sources but also serve as major components of cell membranes. Proteins have a major structural role in animals–most locomotive and organ tissue is protein–and have some work along these lines in plants. However, a major class of proteins called enzymes also has a less popularly appreciated but continuous role as regulators of cellular metabolism, while still other proteins imbed themselves in membranes and act as the cell's gatekeepers. Nucleic acids are overwhelmingly noted for their daily control of the synthesis of proteins and other biochemicals. However, there would be no subsequent generations of cells if nucleic acids did not take the time to replicate themselves during cell division as well.

[Haworth co-indexing entry note]: "Biochemistry and Molecular Biology." Stankus, Tony. Co-published simultaneously in *The Serials Librarian* (The Haworth Press, Inc.) Vol. 27, No. 2/3, 1995, pp. 67-78; and: *Special Format Serials and Issues: Annual Review of . . . , Advances in . . . , Symposia on . . . , Methods in . . .* (ed: Tony Stankus) The Haworth Press, Inc., 1995, pp. 67-78. Single or multiple copies of this article are available from The Haworth Document Delivery Service [1-800-342-9678, 9:00 a.m. - 5:00 p.m. (EST)].

Molecular biology is a field derived from biochemistry. It emphasizes proteins (particularly enzymes and cellular gatekeepers) and nucleic acids. It has achieved an independent status at some institutions, and few life sciences anywhere have not been touched by a "molecularization" of their agenda. It is not unusual, for example, to talk of molecular plant biology or molecular psychiatry. In fields like these, the level of explanation of important life events or behaviors is ideally done in terms of genes encoding for certain proteins. One reads that a given sequence of DNA or RNA encodes for proteins whose cumulation in given cells or tissues lengthens a plant, or perhaps, participates in a cascade of membrane events in neurons that ultimately predisposes an individual toward a behavior. (There are, understandably, greater leaps of scientific faith taken when dealing with human behavior than with plants, but some adherents of the molecular approach ultimately hope to explain both with equal certainty.)

The field of biotechnology is an especially prominent kind of applied molecular biology. It has shown many recent successes, particularly in the food and drug fields. Here again, the stress is most often on the special interplay of nucleic acids and proteins. In many forms of biotechnology, a promising protein is isolated from a microbe, plant, or animal. This leads to an intermediate step of characterizing the nucleic acid sequences that code for that protein. Once the sequence is known, copies containing this sequence are multiplied, often by a technique known as the polymerase chain reaction (PCR). The sequence is inserted into the nucleic acids of a lab culture of cells or microorganisms, or more occasionally into those of a living plant or an animal. In a strategy born of the infective behavior of viruses (which are fundamentally strands of nucleic acids with little more than a protein coat), the inserted nucleic acid sequence begins to express itself within the cells of the host, causing a further multiplication of the desired protein. The protein is then extracted from the cells of the host and purified.

The molecular biology sections of this chapter will deal mostly with the initial characterization of proteins and the segments of associated nucleic acids that directed their individual synthesis, much more so than bulk production. Bulk production will be treated in the chapter on microbiology, the most common partner of molecular biology in biotechnology ventures today. (It is perhaps telling that while there used to be much more fear of runaway mutant germs, there are today few "yeast rights" organizations, as it were, that might picket one's laboratory vats.)

## REVIEWS IN BIOCHEMISTRY AND MOLECULAR BIOLOGY IN MULTISCIENCE JOURNALS

Reviews of biochemistry and molecular biology are constant in the major multiscience journals. *Science, Nature, Cell,* and the *FASEB Journal* typically have one or more in each month's worth of issues. The standing of these reviews in this professional community is very high and comparable to those within the leading journals devoted solely to biochemical reviews. Few libraries serving biochemists could survive without subscriptions to each of these four multiscience journals.

Yet another multispecialty source of frequent reviews is *BioEssays* from the Company of Biologists. Two thirds of the journal is either regular state-of-the-art reviews, or minireviews, and at least half of these are of interest to molecular biologists. There is also a "Roots" column which is essentially a life-and-times review vehicle.

## SOURCES DEVOTED TO REVIEWS IN BIOCHEMISTRY AND MOLECULAR BIOLOGY

Biochemistry and molecular biology have several review serials. The leader among them is the *Annual Review of Biochemistry* from the not-for-profit Annual Reviews, Inc. It follows the standardized format of largely state-of-the-art surveys, although a life-and-times piece on a biochemical pioneer, often autobiographical, is generally found in the begining. It is indispensible in even the smallest library, and this hefty hardbound is among the biggest bargains in science librarianship.

The *Annual Review* is most closely challenged today by *Trends in Biochemical Sciences* from Elsevier. The readability of *Trends* tutorial pieces constitutes the journal's *forte*, and compensates substantially for its steep price. This is the review vehicle of second choice for all libraries.

Choices beyond this depend largely on whether the audience is composed of a broad array of biochemists, or is focused on molecular biology. In the first instance, one might next select *Critical Reviews in Biochemistry and Molecular Biology* from CRC Press. Despite its inclusive-sounding name, its emphasis is still more on the former (biochemistry topics) than on the latter (molecular biology). A softbound bimonthly, it has among the longest state-of-the-art surveys in the field. An alternative worth exploring in institutions with many undergraduate biochemists is the announced revival of the (British) Biochemical Society's *Essays in Biochemistry.* This serial's tutorial style actually preceded that of *Trends*, but the *Essays* were discontinued for over a decade, and only now are reappearing as handy, roughly annual paperbacks that tend to be treated as monographs in many libraries, owing to their ISBNs. The series is quite inexpensive, and will help many a specialist outside his or her niche, even in institutions where there is no undergraduate instruction.

Further selections for a diversified group of biochemists would include some category-of-biochemical reviews. Academic Press is dominant in this area, and its hardbound volumes tend to appear roughly annually, and feature lengthy state-of-the-art reviews. Occasionally, a whole volume will be thematic, and may also contain a life-and-times review of a figure important to the theme. Important members of the Academic review family include *Advances in Carbohydrate Chemistry and Biochemistry, Advances in Lipid Research, Advances in Protein Chemistry,* and *Progress in Nucleic Acids Research and Molecular Biology.* Collections with a somewhat strong stress on lipids may also wish to take *Progress in Lipid Research*, a quarterly with exhaustive surveys, from Pergamon.

Collections with a strong molecular biology emphasis will follow a different ranking of priorities. Up to now, the sequence would have been pretty clear, but since 1994, some reordering of priorities is now arguable. The choice for molecular biologists, after the *Annual Review of Biochemistry* and *Trends in Biochemistry* have been secured, is still likely to be the *Annual Review of Biophysics and Biomolecular Structure* from the Annual Reviews, Inc. Historically, this would be followed closely by the *Quarterly Review of Biophysics* from Cambridge University Press, with *Advances in Enzymology and Related Areas of Molecular Biology* as their primary Academic Press selection (although the protein and nucleic acids volumes mentioned above would also be entirely appropriate). However, it is roughly at this juncture that a bold new contender has emerged, and ironically, from Academic. *Protein Profile* is a rather unique entry, with roots in the prestigious *Journal of Molecular Biology*. It is spiral bound (so as to lay flat in labs) and offers extremely detailed surveys of virtually all available facts about important families of proteins. Each issue is essentially devoted to a single group, usually explored in a single extended review paper, that includes a great deal more tabular information and methodological detail than is found in most reviews. To some degree this *genre* represents a hybrid between Academic's traditional, lengthy state-of-the-art essays and the same publisher's strengths in methods publishing (which will be surveyed shortly). The reference value of these new items is outstanding, but it is not clear whether Academic will gain new customers through this development, so much as threaten one or the other of its historic lines. Given this potential displacement caused by funding *Protein Profile*, only larger groups may also be able to include *Progress in Biophysics and Molecular Biology* from Pergamon, a softbound bimonthly with lengthy state-of-the-art reviews.

## REVIEWS IN REGULAR BIOCHEMISTRY AND MOLECULAR BIOLOGY JOURNALS

Despite the ubiquity of biochemical and molecular biology reviews in multiscience journals, and the plentitude of serials exclusively focused on reviews in the field, there are still literally dozens of other, multifeature journals that publish biochemistry and molecular biology reviews regularly. The importance of these reviews appears to be roughly proportional to the overall reputation of the journals in which they appear.

Review sources of first rank for a diversified population of biochemists include the minireviews in the *Journal of Biological Chemistry* from the American Society for Biological Chemistry and

Molecular Biology, and the somewhat longer "Perspectives in Biochemistry" within *Biochemistry*, its American Chemical Society rival.

Somewhat behind these in prestige are reviews in other North American publications. Academic has long featured "Invited Papers" in the *Archives of Biochemistry and Biophysics*. These tend to be state-of-the-art surveys, but some life-and-times material is not uncommon. The *Journal of Cellular Biochemistry* from Wiley favors papers, termed "Prospects," that are closer to minireviews, and are aimed at pointing out where new work might lead, based on more recent published findings. Canadians are well served by a trio of survey types in *Biochemistry and Cell Biology*, a National Research Council publication. Full-length material is typically listed as a "Review," minireviews appear as "Commentary," pieces that are often produced in conjunction with some career landmark are under "Memorial Lectures."

The British and Continental community is also amply stocked with regular biochemistry journals that include many review papers. The U.K.'s *Biochemical Journal* has always published reviews in its regular issues, generally of the lengthy state-of-the-art type. In recent years, it has taken to reprinting them in a color-enhanced, hardbound format that is available separately for those who do not subscribe to the parent journal. Its purchase is strongly recommended if *Biochemical Journal* is not already on your racks. Also historically based on British talent, but increasing its American participation, is authorship of minireviews in Pergamon's *Comparative Biochemistry and Physiology B: Comparative Biochemistry and Molecular Biology*. This journal is generally more highly regarded in institutions where there are biochemists and molecular biologists serving in zoology departments.

The Continental scene is crowded with good sources. The Federation of European Biochemical Societies has two major outlets for them: *FEBS Letters* and the *European Journal of Biochemistry*. The *Letters* features two review types: conventional "minireviews" and a "hypothesis" series, the latter allowing for some speculation, much in the manner of the "Prospects" reviews of the U.S. *Journal of Cellular Biochemistry*. The *European Journal of Biochemistry* also features two types: conventional state-of-the-art reviews, and

"Lectures," which may take on either a life-and-times or a tutorial approach.

The queen of European reviewing sources is *Biochimica et Biophysica Acta*, the gargantuan journal from Elsevier. While still available as a consolidated journal subscription, and one containing almost a hundred review papers scattered throughout its many sections each year, *BBA* is also the source of two subsections that particularly highlight reviews. These are *BBA: Reviews on Biomembranes* and *BBA: Reviews on Cancer*. The audience for these sections is less narrow than might be supposed given that membranes are controllers of the incoming and outgoing traffic of biochemicals into cells, and that cancer, as a general theme, probably funds more biochemical research than any other ailment or medical initiative.

There are other, more specialized journals of biochemistry that frequently feature reviews. Similar in membrane slant to the above noted *BBA* section, the lesser known *Journal of Bioenergetics and Biomembranes* from Plenum includes minireviews. The *Journal of Photochemistry and Photobiology* from Elsevier stresses "New Trends Invited Reviews," which have a somewhat personalized "my lab" approach.

Journals devoted to major categories of biochemicals have intermittent reviews. The *Journal of Lipid Research* from Lipid Research, Inc. features lengthy state-of-the-art papers. *Glycoconjugate Journal*, a title based on compounds that have a significant carbohydrate portion, has minireviews termed "Glycopinions." Life and times pieces are found in the traditional leader, the *International Journal for Peptide and Protein Research* from Munksgaard under the aegis of "Historical Perspectives." That source, however, may be overshadowed by the number and diversity of reviews in *Protein Science*, a Cambridge University Press publication that offers a special break to members of the American Society for Biological Chemistry and Molecular Biology, the publishers of the *Journal of Biological Chemistry*. It has not only a life and times "Recollections," series, but conventional state-of-the-art reviews, and award lectures. The *Journal of Protein Chemistry* from Plenum is about third place as a source of reviews, largely invited minireviews. *Nucleic Acids Research* from Oxford University Press has extended

"Survey and Summary" papers that have both state-of-the-art and installment review characteristics.

The molecular biology contingent will seek out reviews in the major general biochemistry journals, the specialized protein and nucleic acids journals, and in three molecular biology journals. These three are, in rough order of the importance of their reviews: the *EMBO Journal* from Oxford University Press (the EMBO Medal Research Review, life-and-times); *Molecular Biology Reports* from Kluwer (minireviews); and the *European Biophysical Journal* from Springer ("Invited Reviews," state-of-the-art with life-and-times detail not unusual). Most molecular biologists also scan journals of microbiology, especially those specializing in virology, for reviews. Cell biology titles are likely to be on their reading lists as well.

## THEME AND SYMPOSIA LITERATURE IN BIOCHEMISTRY AND MOLECULAR BIOLOGY

American biochemists meet frequently, and in the thousands at a time. The full text of these talks is understandably rarely published in any one place. Rather, it appears that most of the major talks get placed individually in a wide variety of outlets. The *FASEB Journal* remains the leader in their publication, with 50% of its full-text content derived from conference presentations reworked into brief reviews, and up to 10,000 abstracts as well. In recent years, the *Journal of Cellular Biochemistry* has been catching up, with both abstracts coverage and selected full-text of major talks of the Keystone Symposia, a series of forums organized annually in the Rockies and on the West Coast.

In certain respects, molecular biologists have it even better. Their agenda has come to dominate one of the few full-text biological symposia series in the U.S., the *Cold Spring Harbor Symposia on Quantitative Biology* from Cold Spring Harbor Press. This series is famed not only for its editor, Nobel Laureate and institute director, James Watson, but for its candid photos of conference participants enjoying themselves during concurrent social events. While neither biochemistry nor molecular biology could be safely said to dominate another irregular periodical, the *Annals of the New York Acade-*

*my of Sciences*, enough of that multidisciplinary series is pertinent to make its adoption in larger institutions strongly suggested.

The Continental Europeans and the British have a brisk trade in scientific conferences for biochemists and molecular biologists. Few publications cover so many so fully as the *Biochemical Society Transactions*. While most of these are confined to meetings held in the UK, a rather large number of honorary, dedicatory or invited lectures and awards ceremonies are also covered, making it one of the better life-and-times resources for internationally important biochemists, regardless of their permanent affiliations. Molecular biology conferences in the UK are not as routinely well covered. However, Kluwer's *Molecular Biology Reports,* via its "Workshops" papers, handles more than most other sources, and includes many Continental gatherings as well. On the Continent, *Biochimie*, now an Elsevier publication, has special issues for meetings of French biochemists, while *Biological Chemistry, Hoppe-Seyler* from Dr. Gruyter, handles them for the Germans.

Certain categories of biochemicals have their own conferences. *Carbohydrate Research* from Elsevier, the *Journal of Steroid Chemistry and Biochemistry* from Pergamon, and the *Journal of Lipid Research* from Lipid Research Inc., all feature meetings issues, many with full-text papers.

## *METHODS LITERATURE IN BIOCHEMISTRY AND MOLECULAR BIOLOGY*

Highly novel methods papers are accepted in most of the major journals of biochemistry and molecular biology. However, even some fairly significant improvements or workable variants on previously published methods appear less welcome. In other cases, particularly useful adaptations are hidden as trade secrets from a wider readership as their scientific discoverers become entrepreneurs or join established biotech businesses. Fortunately, there are some outstanding serials which see value in reporting ongoing improvements in techniques, and are of such status that even for-profit scientists view publication there as an "advertisement" of their firm's prowess.

Standing at the pinnacle is *Analytical Biochemistry* from Academic Press. The "analytical" portion of the title is reminiscent of the first (and one of the continuing) tasks of biochemical methodology: isolation and identification of biochemical components. While not abandoning this valuable work, *Analytical Biochemistry* has become far more wide-ranging topically and includes a wide variety of manipulative and tailoring techniques. At a substantial distance behind in terms of prestige for general biochemists is Dekker's *Preparative Biochemistry*. Its cost is but a fraction of the better known *Analytical Biochemistry*, and is well worth acquiring for Ph.D. programs, med schools, drug and biotech firms. A surprisingly rising star is the *Journal of Agricultural and Food Chemistry* from the American Chemical Society. Whereas its old content was largely sanitation, nutrition, and pesticides, its new content includes substantial amounts of modern biochemistry and molecular biology. This is reasonable when one steps back and realizes that many food supply improvements are now the results of genetic engineering and that altered plants, in particular, are amenable to bulk production with fewer regulatory restrictions than animal stocks. Moreover, many long established food companies are sufficiently capitalized to branch out in these areas, like biotechnology, which require long term investment before a payoff.

The molecular biology end of this field is extremely well stocked with methods information services. The most venerable of these is a voluminous hardbound series from Academic, *Methods in Enzymology*. Far more inclusive than its title suggests, each thematic volume is a veritable symposia-in-print of discursive papers reviewing the best approaches. It offers biochemists, molecular biologists, and cellular physiologists a great deal of comparative advantage information on given procedures, with specifications as detailed as the best glassware for a given experiment. *Methods in Enzymology* not only reports a great many procedures for the first time in the literature, but it ferrets out and cites the useful methods sections and fine-print footnotes in journals that that are not primarily thought of as emphasizing technique. In recent years, Academic has brought up a companion paperback updating service, called simply *Methods*, that is recommended for the most active collections.

Another approach to keeping up-to-date methodologically has

been Wiley's looseleaf service, *Current Protocols in Molecular Biology*. Here, approximately a dozen major procedures are updated periodically. Key papers that serve as examples of the technique in action are always being added to the references, along with any modifications that have cropped up. *Current Protocols* has the intriguing combination of a largely Boston-Cambridge, MA biomedical authorship (Harvard and its Hospitals; MIT and its Whitehead Institute) and international appeal. It is handier than *Methods in Enzymology* and has almost as much authority when dealing with more common molecular biology procedures.

Bringing up third place is *Biotechniques* from Eaton. While older than *Current Protocols*, it has not made as large an impression on the field. Nonetheless, it belongs in virtually all active molecular biology collections, a prospect that is entirely affordable.

The polymerase chain reaction is probably the most exciting tool developed in molecular biology over the last decade. It is not surprising that a journal is now entirely focused on it, or that powerhouse Cold Spring Harbor publishes it. *PCR Methods and Applications* is clearly the leader in this ever-widening niche of molecular biology.

Certain more traditional techniques, particularly those used in protein structure determination, merit their own sections within established journals if not their own new journals. The venerable *Journal of Molecular Biology* from Academic Press publishes "Crystallization Notes" and "Sequence Notes" largely for those who use X-ray crystallography. Another veteran, *Nucleic Acids Research* from Oxford University Press, publishes a great deal of reference data under three recurring features entitled "For the Record," "Sequences," and "Methods."

Three newer titles tend towards the biotechnology end of the field, but are still of substantial methodological interest for basic scientists. *Proteins* from Wiley is clearly the most academic, and the journal of first choice. *Protein Engineering* from Oxford is somewhat more applied, and recommended as a second choice. It has a lengthier pedigree than the newest entry *Protein Expression and Purification* from Academic, which, given that firm's excellence in methods reporting, will likely be worth examining more closely.

Two new journals have a strong interest in peptide methodology.

(Peptides are the building blocks of proteins.) While it is still too early to rank one over the other, readers of Munksgaard's *International Journal of Peptide and Protein Research*, a traditional leader in peptides, in particular, will want to track both Bentham's *Protein and Peptide Letters*, and Wiley's *Journal of Peptide Science*.

Finally, the naming of complex biochemicals and the terminology of molecular biology have become so complicated that access to "nomenclatural" literature is becoming more and more important. While a number of European biochemical journals, including *Biochimica et Biophysica Acta* have historically offered reviews of new compounds and their naming, the *European Journal of Biochemistry* from Springer has come to lead in this service.

# Cell Biology

The cell occupies the same role in 20th century biology that the rat had in the 19th century lab: the most important living thing upon which to try experiments. While it may share this limelight with certain bacteria, just about everything smaller than a cell (viruses, proteins, nucleic acids, drugs) is deliberately introduced into cell cultures today. Moreover, virtually everything larger than a cell is ground up at some stage of the experiment into cells or cell fractions. This makes special genre serials in cell biology important to a community that is larger than those who call themselves cell biologists. It is important to note that the field has historically evolved from two important constituencies. The first were those who microscopically analysed its internal structures and enveloping membranes: the cytologists. The medical specialty of anatomic pathology is still highly dependent on their findings. The second were those who kept cell cultures ingeniously alive for various experiments in physiology and pharmacology: the cellular physiologists. There are persistent traces of these two interest groups in many review, symposia, and methods serials today.

## REVIEWS OF CELL BIOLOGY IN MULTISCIENCE JOURNALS

Since cells have been so central to the pursuit of modern laboratory biology, reviews in cell biology are very common in the major multiscience journals. *Science* from the American Association for the Advancement of Science, and *Nature*, handled by Pergamon for

---

[Haworth co-indexing entry note]: "Cell Biology." Stankus, Tony. Co-published simultaneously in *The Serials Librarian* (The Haworth Press, Inc.) Vol. 27, No. 2/3, 1995, pp. 79-86; and: *Special Format Serials and Issues: Annual Review of . . . , Advances in . . . , Symposia on . . . , Methods in . . .* (ed: Tony Stankus) The Haworth Press, Inc., 1995, pp. 79-86. Single or multiple copies of this article are available from The Haworth Document Delivery Service [1-800-342-9678, 9:00 a.m. - 5:00 p.m. (EST)].

the British Association, are paramount sources. Within the life sciences generally, the *FASEB Journal* from the Federation of American Societies for Experimental Biology, *Bioessays* from Cambridge on behalf of the (British) Company of Biologists, and, unsurprisingly, *Cell* have important reviews. (*Cell* can, with justice, be classified as either one of the most important multiscience journals, or as the leading journal of cell biology.) The range of length of text and number of references goes from the minireview in *Cell* and in *Bioessays* through the mid-range in *Science* and *Nature*, with the longest appearing in the *FASEB Journal*. The style in most of these journals is state-of-the-art, but *Bioessays* has a recurring "Roots" section with life-and-times papers as well. Modestly-toned, life-and-times reviews also can be found in the edited versions of the Nobel Prize speeches reprinted in *Science*. *Cell*'s minireviews, by contrast, are famously provocative.

## REVIEWS OF CELL BIOLOGY
## IN NEIGHBORING DISCIPLINES

Journals with frequent reviews of cell biology are also found in the literature of physiology, biochemistry, and developmental biology. The *Annual Review of Physiology* features medium length cellular physiology surveys, with *Physiological Reviews* having very long essays. The state-of-the art approach is the most common in both, although some life-and-times papers routinely appear as introductions in the *Annual Review of Physiology*. Reviews on cell membranes are frequently featured in *Biochimica et Biophysica Acta's* special section: *Reviews on Biomembranes*. Most of its reviews are traditional, lengthy, state-of-the-art works. *Anatomy and Embryology* from Springer is the leader in descriptive microanatomy among developmental sources of reviews, mixing state-of-the-art with a fair amount of life-and-times papers. *Acta Anatomica* from Karger has occasional supplements devoted to exceptionally lengthy reviews, with the same format mix as *Anatomy and Embryology.*

All the physiology journals mentioned in this section are automatic choices in most life sciences collections, and would therefore cause no added cost for the collector of reviews. *Biochimica et Biophysica Acta* is a titanically expensive exception. Its "Biomembranes" review section is available for separate purchase and is recommended where the comprehensive subscription cannot be afforded. The option of adding the microscopic anatomy and developmental titles is dependent on local emphases. Those titles are somewhat more expensive than most of the physiology sources, although still cheaper than *Biochimica et Biophysica Acta.*

## REVIEWS IN CELL BIOLOGY JOURNALS

A number of leading cell biology journals feature reviews. Their number has appeared to increase since the highly successful introduction of minireviews in *Cell.* Medium sized, traditional reviews are present but still relatively infrequent in the *Journal of Cell Biology.* By contrast, a mix containing state-of-the-art and tutorial minireviews has become quite common in the form of "Commentaries" in the *Journal of Cell Science* from the (British) Company of Biologists. (That journal is also becoming a leader in the use of color for both research and tutorial reasons in their illustrations.) *Experimental Cell Research* from Academic features an irregular series of "Special Articles and Reviews."

An important journal covering a somewhat more specialized area within cell biology, the *Journal of Cellular Biochemistry,* from Liss-Wiley, occasionally publishes papers specifically designed to discuss agenda-setting. These reviews are termed "Prospects," and generally have a state-of-the-art approach. These papers contain a good deal of frank advocacy whereby review authors explain why they feel a given theme or technique will become increasingly important.

Once again, virtually all of these journals are already in any decent cell biology collection: no added expenditure is necessary to gain access to their reviews.

## SERIALS SPECIFICALLY DEVOTED TO CELL BIOLOGY REVIEWS

In a reversal of the usual pattern of review serial development, the *Annual Reviews* foundation belatedly followed the success of a longstanding for-profit entry: the *International Review of Cytology* from Academic Press. The *International Review* was founded in 1952 by Bourne and Danielli, two early pioneers in cell physiology and cell membrane studies, respectively. It started as a hardbound annual with a strong mix of papers of both life-and-times and state-of-the-art style. The life-and-times papers sought to reinforce and codify the academic lineage of cell biology, arguing that it was no longer just a stepchild of anatomy or physiology, but a discipline in its own right. The state-of-the-art papers denoted the need to comparatively evaluate many new laboratory approaches, a sign of a vitally busy field. Today, the *International Review*'s papers are arguably the lengthiest in cell biology. They cover the widest variety of cell types and are known for the rather more exotic animal and plant sources of those cells. The *International Review*'s reference lists regularly range into the hundreds per paper. The *International Review* has adopted the subtitle *A Survey of Cell Biology* denoting its encyclopedic scope. It features "theme-review" issues from time to time, so that it is literally possible to find hundreds of pages with thousands of references on a single type of cell or concept in cellular biology. There are as many as four physical volumes of the *International Review* each year, although two or three volumes are more common.

The ongoing transformation of the *International Review* from a conventional annual through its addition of extra volumes and its enhanced discussion may have been accelerated by the arrival of the *Annual Review of Cell Biology* in 1985, and *Trends in Cell Biology* in 1991. This *Annual Review* exploded onto the scene and has effectively taken over the medium-length state-of-the-art paper. It also emphasizes more mainstream topics than the *International Review*. Ironically, this *Annual Review* is one of the few of its foundational family with virtually no life-and-times papers. (The fact that the *Annual Review of Physiology* already does this for some cellular physiologists may have something to do with it.) *Trends in Cell Biology* combines state-of-the-art minireviews with nice tutorial papers. Readability is one of its classic strengths, and it tends to undercut the venerable *International Review* in undergraduate collections. Both the *Annual Review* and *Trends in Cell Biology* now represent better choices for most collections, but no graduate, medical school, or biotechnology programs should be without the *International Review*.

A number of more specialized reviews also exist. The leading example is Academic's *Current Topics in Cellular Regulation*. This hardbound review stands at the intersection of those who view themselves as cellular "maintenance" physiologists and those with a view towards tinkering with the cell's normal function by identifying nucleic acids and proteins that alter the day-to-day functioning of the cell and thereby initiate new events in the cell's life cycle. As with the *International Review*, the papers are generally traditional: long, comprehensive, and extensively referenced. This series is particularly recommended for a cell biology community that coordinates with a molecular biology or pharmacology group.

## SYMPOSIA AND THEME ISSUES IN CELL BIOLOGY

The *Annals of the New York Academy of Sciences* publishes several volumes of live symposia annually, with topics of interest to cell biology treated in one or two numbers. The *Ciba Foundation Symposia*, a largely English language series sponsored by a Swiss consortium, also devotes about one in ten of its irregular symposia volumes to cellular topics. Both of these occasionally relevant outlets–indeed most librarians would do better to buy the pertinent issues individually–must hold a secondary place, however, to at least three other symposia and theme entries, with a few others yet challenging.

The first of these, the *Cold Spring Harbor Symposia on Quantitative Biology*, covers a wide variety of topics in molecular biology, virology, immunology, and biotechnology, topics of high interest to cell biologists. The *Cold Spring Harbor Symposia* is arguably the most star-studded of any life sciences series. The laboratory that hosts the series is on Long Island and is directed by Nobel Laureate James Watson. It is also among the most physically substantial (all the talks are printed full-length) and comes in one or more hardbound volumes annually. Among other human interest features, one finds many highly informal pictures of the participants, generally in Bermuda shorts–appropriate to this sometimes resort area–and smiling for the camera.

While the *Cold Spring Harbor* series is of world importance, two other geographic constituencies have strong competitor symposia. What might be called the California school of cell physiology has long published within the *Journal of Cellular Physiology* its UCLA symposium proceedings. This series has recently obtained the even greater support of a newly organized "Keystone" foundation, composed largely of major western U.S. universities, research institutes, and corporate sponsors, and may one day challenge the *Cold Spring Harbor* series. It has the continuing disadvantage of primarily featuring paragraph-sized abstracts of the oral presentations, as opposed to their full text, in most cases. The full text of presentations is featured, however, in a Supplement series of the *Journal of Cell Science*. Its authorship is largely British, and its format is very attractively hardbound. It is not clear that these roughly annual "symposia" always involve live presentations. (Some may be after-the-fact submissions.) These supplements may well be "theme" issues in some cases, but it is clear, once again, that the excellent reproductions and increasing use of color within them provide a competitive advantage. Not surprisingly, the publisher, the Company of Biologists, offers these theme supplements for sale to those who do not take a subscription to the *Journal of Cell Science*, and these do a brisk business.

The combination of review-style articles focusing on a single theme is also common in a bimonthly softbound series from Saunders, *Seminars in Cell Biology*, a journal featuring a mix of traditional and minireviews. This series, despite a modest price, has not, however, made as large an impact as might be expected. By contrast, the somewhat more-specialized *Current Topics in Membranes and Transport*, a highly traditional hardbound appearing once or twice a year from Academic, is a must purchase for all collections that involve either the cell physiology or cell microanatomy constituencies of the field. It should be noted that "transport" in the cell biology context means the traffic of drugs or naturally occuring substances through the various gates in the cell membrane. This is a linking of concepts that goes back to the initial interests of Bourne and Danielli, Academic's pioneering editors in hardbound review serials.

Selection in this group offers relatively limited added costs. The

*Cold Spring Harbor* series is the title of first choice for those who can afford less than the full complement.

## METHODS SERIALS IN CELL BIOLOGY

Keeping all those cells alive outside a living body is not any easy task, and not only do cells from differing organisms require differing techniques, but differing types of cells from the same body require them as well. The longstanding leader in this field has been the Tissue Culture Association. "Tissues" in this context means islands of cultured cells that are related by the job they do within a body or the site of their origin. These tissues are generally kept alive in nutrient broths or in gelatins maintained in petri dishes or test tubes, a situation termed "in vitro" (in laboratory glassware). Two serials from the Tissue Culture Association cover this area. Both the nominally more sophisticated *In Vitro–Cellular and Developmental Biology* from this association and its more honestly named *Journal of Tissue Culture Methods* are essentials for extensive practical observations and comparisons of techniques. Critics have suggested rather pompously that the TCA is the society for mere technicians–a cavalier attitude about which the TCA seems highly defensive and which is behind the revamping of *In Vitro*. It might be noted, nonetheless, that the new *In Vitro* is still tremendously involved with methods, and has more recently taken full advantage of the upsurge of interest into plant cell work as a result of rosey prospects for success in agricultural biotechnology. From time to time the Association also revises its *TCA Manual*, another practical work, with something like a *Handbuch* approach.

The more "conceptually oriented" organization in the field, the American Society for Cell Biology, has also been cognizant of the needs for methods information. The ASCB has wisely chosen to co-opt a hardbound series originally begun by Prescott, a leading cell physiologist, rather than starting an entirely new series of their own. In doing so, they have continued to cooperate with Academic Press, so that Prescott's *Methods in Cell Physiology* is now *Methods in Cell Biology*. Most of the papers are fairly brief minireviews of a highly instructive tutorial nature. This methods series is a worthy companion to TCA publications and belongs even in the more moderately sized collections.

There are a number of competing or complementary regularly issued journals. At this time, they are of less general need but important to given constituencies. *Stain Technology*, a Williams and Wilkins softbound, focuses on the special dyes necessary to visualize cell structures or cell transformations under powerful microscopes. This is a traditional concern of medical school microanatomy and pathology, since diseased cells, such as those seen in cancer biopsies, often have diagnostic staining patterns. More engineering oriented are a number of journals focused on biological microscopy in general. These include Liss-Wiley's *Cytometry*, and the *Journal of Microscopy* from Blackwell.

There are two relative newcomers to the well-established cell methods field. One offers greater liveliness, the other offers enhanced perspectives through more formal reviews. Somewhat broader in interest and more directly competitive with the TCA's *In Vitro* and the *Journal of Tissue Culture Methods*, is *Methods in Molecular and Cellular Biology* from Wiley-Liss, managers of the important *Journal of Cellular Physiology* and the *Journal of Cellular Biochemistry*. It is a softbound bimonthly whose impact has not yet been clear, but whose presence is a demonstration of the extraordinary interest in practical details. Given the plethora of contributions in these more regularly issued journals of methods, it is not surprising that, once again, Academic has weighed in with another hardbound series, the roughly annual *Advances in Cell Culture*. The papers here are uniformly longer than those found in *Methods in Cell Biology* and are generally more discursive and comparative. Nonetheless, *Methods in Cell Biology* is still a better first choice for offering more topics in addition to straightforward culture alone. It should be noted that cell membranes have their own methods review, the irregular hardbound from Plenum, *Cell Membranes: Methods and Reviews*. This is a title primarily for strong subspecialty collections.

A minimal strategy in a tight fiscal climate is a combination of *In Vitro* and *Methods in Cell Biology*. They have a seniority of reputation and a wider scope than any of the other titles mentioned. Most of those titles cost substantially less, however, than subscriptions to the regular journals for cellular research that they so ably supplement.

# Drugs and Poisons

The making of medicines and the monitoring of their absorption and effects has an amazingly balkanized occupational history. This has led to a plethora of journals, with a tremendous need for reviews, particularly for those that cross over from their originating segment of the field and inform other segments of the drug and poison community. Let us list some of the main groups with an interest in the field.

*First*, we have the people who discover drugs in their primitive or natural state. They have often been trained initially as botanists or anthropologists. Their journal titles typically involve phrases such as "ethnobotany," "pharmacognoscy," or "natural products," or "ethnopharmacology."

*Second*, we have the people who make the essential ingredients of drugs synthetically in the lab. They often aim to replicate or tailor natural products. They are, nonetheless, organic chemists by initial training, and advance to a status as medicinal chemists. Most of the journals that deal with this group are styled "medicinal chemistry."

*Third*, we have the people who prescribe drugs. They are licensed physicians, most often primary care doctors and psychiatrists. As a practical matter, their core literatures will not be reviewed here. Psychopharmacology and neurology reviews will be discussed in a separate chapter on neuroscience, while selected reviews of internal medicine are covered in a chapter devoted to physiology.

*Fourth*, we have the people who dispense drugs. They are pharmacists (except in the U.K. where they are, confusingly enough, referred to as "chemists"). The journals that most pharmacists read

[Haworth co-indexing entry note]: "Drugs and Poisons." Stankus, Tony. Co-published simultaneously in *The Serials Librarian* (The Haworth Press, Inc.) Vol. 27, No. 2/3, 1995, pp. 87-102; and: *Special Format Serials and Issues: Annual Review of . . . , Advances in . . . , Symposia on . . . , Methods in . . .* (ed: Tony Stankus) The Haworth Press, Inc., 1995, pp. 87-102. Single or multiple copies of this article are available from The Haworth Document Delivery Service [1-800-342-9678, 9:00 a.m. - 5:00 p.m. (EST)].

are termed "pharmaceutical." These deal partly with the retail or hospital-based dispensing of drugs in their finished form, along with suitable patient advisory at the point of sale or distribution to administering nurses. But mostly, pharmaceutical journals report on progress in turning the essential ingredients of drugs–supplied by the medicinal chemists and prescribed by the doctors–into convenient, consistent, unspoiled dosages of medicines: pills, capsules, syrups, injections, etc., long before the medicines ever get to the pharmacy or clinic.

*Fifth*, we have the people who most systematically study the pathways and intended effects of drugs after their ingestion. They are pharmacologists, and their journals are termed "pharmacological."

*Sixth*, we have the people who study the untoward effects of drugs or other agents brought into the body through the environment. They are toxicologists, and their journals are called "toxicological." (Poisons that cause genetic defects will be dealt with in a separate chapter on genes and development.)

*Seventh*, we note that a good deal of the preliminary design of drugs seems to be the work of computer graphics experts. It is not unusual to see phrases such as "computer" or "molecular graphics" in their reporting outlets.

*Eighth*, we have various patent and oversight bodies, composed of virtually all of these constituencies mentioned thus far, with the addition of public health officials, epidemiologists, statisticians, and sometimes attorneys and politicians. Most of their publications will be termed "regulatory."

This chapter will make mention of all the specialties to some degree, but most strongly focuses on the pharmacologist as the central coordinator of all these diverse guilds.

While it is clearly understood that in the U.S. MDs go to medical school, the overwhelming majority of dispensing pharmacists go to separate, largely bachelor-degree-granting schools of pharmacy that are not attached to medical schools. Schools of pharmacy are more closely tied to programs resembling those in university departments of chemistry. Pharmacologists and most toxicologists are usually graduate degree holders. Although some MDs take advanced training in pharmacology or toxicology, most drug and poison scientists today have backgrounds in pharmacy or chemistry to start with. Within the U.S., however, most pharmacologists cannot experiment on humans without the cooperation of MDs. The subtitle "clinical" in a name of a journal tends to indicate that work on humans–and therefore involving at least some MDs–as opposed to work on monkeys, dogs, rats, etc., is being featured. Conversely, titles which use the word "pharmaceutics" tend to be concerned at least as much with the composition of the drug–involving both pharmacists and medicinal chemists–as they are with lab animals or patients. These are not infallible distinctions but lead to an explanation of the author's differing recommendations.

When making recommendations in this chapter, the author uses the term "undergraduate" or "smallest" for bachelor-degree-granting schools of pharmacy or liberal arts college chemistry departments that have a number of synthetic organic or natural products chemists.

"Intermediate" collections are those at departments of chemistry that offer master's degrees in medicinal chemistry or pharmacy schools with masters in pharmacology or toxicology.

Other intermediate collections, usually designated as "intermediate clinical," may be at hospitals which employ several pharmacists and pharmacologists, but which do not maintain a large formal program in pharmacology.

"Comprehensive" or the "largest" collections are taken to mean the largest medical schools, schools of any type with a Ph.D. program in a pharmacology discipline, and the principal research and development centers for drug companies.

Fortunately, the trend towards subspecialization of the drug field by category of organ system (e.g., the cardiovascular system) or by given category of disease (e.g., cancer) or drug target (e.g., viruses) is not yet entirely out of control. Pharmacology is still dominated by more general journals, although the major killer diseases (heart, cancer, and infection) have a few prominent titles each. The most glaring exceptions are drug journals for diseases of the nervous system, or for coping with emotional crises. Neuropharmacology and psychopharmacology are vast fields and increasingly separated from the literature of "somatic" pharmacology. (Once again, the reader is reminded that these topics and their literature will be treated in the neurosciences chapter.)

The simplification of serials recommendations is, however, frustrated by the far-flung geography of competitive pharmacology powers, and even of pharmacology publishers. Leadership by American firms such as Eli Lilly; SmithKline and Beckman, and Merck, Sharp, and Dohme, is hotly contested by British firms like Glaxo, Burroughs-Wellcome, and ICI, Swiss firms such as Sandoz and CIBA-Geigy, and so on, leading to continued support of many national journals of pharmacology. Even New Zealand will be shown to be a particulary prominent publishing source. Legal drugs cross national boundaries and oceans almost as readily as illegal ones. Internationally, there is so much money in the drug business and so many layers of scientists, physicians, businessmen, and governmental regulators that advertising revenues fuel the creation of many new serial titles aimed at each step of the trade. There are literally hundreds of journals in pharmacology and its cognate sciences, and most of them, from time-to-time, accept reviews or symposia. The drug companies themselves frequently underwrite the research leading to reviews or the holding of scientific congresses with the underlying idea that this investment in research and publication will accelerate the acceptance process for new drugs they wish to market. The acceptance of a single new drug can yield hundreds of millions of dollars for its firm. Nonetheless, the goal of this chapter is not so much to list all drug journals, subsidized or otherwise, as to indicate which of the better journals feature solid reviews, symposia, or methods material on a fairly regular basis.

## *REVIEWS IN PHARMACOLOGY AND RELATED FIELDS IN MORE GENERAL JOURNALS*

The revamped *FASEB* Journal from the Federation of American Societies for Experimental Biology has taken over from *Science* and *Nature* leadership in presenting the most significant pharmacology reviews to the general scientific and biomedical community. These reviews are generally of a middle length (10 double columned pages and 50-100 references) and are state-of-the-art in style and intent. Pharmacology reviews are presented alongside those in cell biology, physiology, nutrition, immunology, and other fields with which drug sciences are increasingly intermeshed. The *FASEB Journal* is the first round selection of a general science title for pharmacologists. Of course, virtually no science library could function without *Science* and *Nature*, but duplication and routing policy may suggest a surprisingly lower status for them than for *FASEB*.

There are two other more general science titles with valuable reviews for pharmacologists. *Life Sciences* from Pergamon is a vehicle designed for rapid preliminary communications in a number of the more molecularized biological disciplines, and publishes hundreds of "letter-size" papers in a year. However, it is rapidly gaining at least as much status for dozens of its "minireviews," many of which are pharmacological. It has the next priority in general science journal selection for intermediate or larger clinical collections but may be omitted in some undergraduate pharmacy and chemistry collections. Finally, a hardbound irregular from Springer designed for three specialties, the *Review of Physiology, Biochemistry, and Pharmacology* has a solid history and moderate current reputation. It belongs primarily in doctoral level pharmacology institutions and most medical schools.

## *REVIEWS IN PHARMACOLOGY AND RELATED FIELDS IN MORE SPECIALIZED JOURNALS*

Pharmacology is also well served by an assortment of review serials aimed specifically at the pharmacological community. No less than six general pharmacology titles contend for review leadership. Patterns of preference are connected with scientific and publishing geopolitics. There are linkages between the sources that pharmacologists favor for their reviews and those they favor for their original research article reading. These are often bonds of shared publisher, shared professional society, or shared geography.

To a substantial degree, those societies or for-profit publishers that feature a journal exclusively for reviews tend to have fewer full-length state-of-the-art review sections within other journals that they field, although minireviews and life-and-times pieces will still be common. If a worthy, lengthy state-of-the-art paper is sent to one of their journals for original search, it is often referred to the related journal for reviews.

The most exhaustive surveys are found in *Pharmacological Reviews* from the American Society for Pharmacology and Experimental Therapeutics. It is a quarterly softbound, distributed by Williams and Wilkins, principally on behalf of the American Society for Pharmacology and Experimental Therapeutics, but with the cooperation of British and Scandinavian societies as well. It is the favorite review source of readers of the *Journal of Pharmacology and Experimental Therapeutics* (U.S.), the *British Journal of Pharmacology*, and a number of Scandinavian titles. Somewhat more compact essays are to be found in the *Annual Reviews of Pharmacology and Toxicology* from the not-for-profit Annual Reviews, Inc., another largely American vehicle. Both of these U.S.-based sources stress state-of-the-art work, although the papers in *Annual Review* occasionally include life-and-times pieces. Both of these pharmacology leaders are reasonably priced and are recommended for even the smallest undergraduate collections.

A third title, *Advances in Pharmacology*, is from Academic and is characteristic of its genre: very lengthy state-of-the-art essays issued roughly annually in a hardbound format. It is a good choice for intermediate libraries, both clinical and pharmaceutical.

The British, despite their primary support of *Pharmacological Reviews*, have two additional vehicles for lengthy state-of-the-art reviews. Both feature some Anglo-American cooperation. *Medicinal Research Reviews* features an American publisher, Wiley, with a strong contingent of largely UK authors. Pergamon counters with *Pharmacology and Therapeutics*, with an American Editor-in-Chief and a majority of British contributors. *Medicinal Research Reviews*, a bimonthly, is only moderately more expensive than *Pharmacological Reviews*, and deserves a higher priority than the Pergamon entry. *Pharmacology and Therapeutics* appears twice as often, but costs about three times as much. It is recommended for the largest collections. While it might appear that *Medicinal Research Reviews* is heavily slanted towards synthetic chemistry or pharmaceutics, its scope is broader than the title suggests. It is recommended for intermediate collections, including clinical ones.

The Continental scene features four rivals. One is a choice for even the smallest collections, one is recommended for intermediate collections, two are suitable primarily for comprehensive pharmacology collections. Elsevier has a winner in its *Trends in Pharmacological Sciences*. It stands in sharp contrast in approach to its rivals. Its monthly minireview papers are arguably the most lively and most current of any review source, surpassing even those in *Life Sciences*. Many of them are indeed tutorial without in any sense being trivial, and are accompanied by helpful illustrations that are not characteristic of most other review sources. Its fairly steep price is its only drawback, a disadvantage it shares with its titanic companion Elsevier journal for original research, the *European Journal of Pharmacology*. Nonetheless, *Trends* is recommended for even the smallest collections owing to its exceptional innovativeness.

Tradition demands mention of three other Continental entries in the review field. They are representative of the exceptionally powerful Swiss and German pharmaceutical communities, and a handful of strong publishers: Cantor, Birkhauser, Springer and Karger.

*Progress in Drug Research*, a review serial from the Swiss-German firm Birkhauser, is geoscientifically related to another Swiss-German journal for original research from Cantor, *Arzneimittelforschung*. *Progress* was originally entitled *Fortschritte der Arzneimittelforschung*. Although this Birkhauser entry is now very largely in English, it has been a favorite of German-speaking Europe, whose principal outlets have also included Birkhauser's *Agents and Actions* and Springer's *Naunyn-Schmiedebergs Archives of Pharmacology*. *Progress in Drug Research* might be regarded as a modern day central European *Jahrbuch*, and is recommended for intermediate pharmaceutical collections.

Two other somewhat irregular hardbound series are generally devoted to collections of reviews, but sometimes include symposia, or at times even a single book-length treatment. Both *Progress in Basic and Clinical Pharmacology* and *Progress in Biochemical Pharmacology* are from Karger. Both a high price and a diminished current standing make them optional titles for all but the largest collections.

There are a number of other review journals that are more specialized. *Natural Products Reports*, a monthly softbound, from the Royal (U.K.) Society of Chemistry, is the leading review source for its field. It belongs in every medicinal chemistry and pharmacognoscy collection, and many ethnobotany or plant biochemistry ones as well.

Another title appeals strongly to the organic chemists within the field and is U.S.-based. Academic fields a softbound *Annual Reports in Medicinal Chemistry* that is sponsored, but not published by, a division of the American Chemical Society. It has both state-of-the-art and installment reviews of intermediate length. While optional for intermediate clinical libraries, it is a first choice for schools of pharmacy and most university departments with a large group of synthetic or natural products chemists. A second choice, *Progress in Medicinal Chemistry* from Elsevier, has somewhat less impact, and is a good backup for this audience.

*Advances in Drug Research* is another in Academic's hardbound series. Appearing on a roughly annual basis, and featuring long state-of-the-art essays, it is marketed primarily for schools of pharmacy. It is also a good choice for programs in medicinal chemistry.

Surveys of devices and procedures for drug delivery, including both innovative means of encapsulating oral medications as well as perfusion pumps, implantable sponges, time-release devices, etc., are found in *Critical Reviews of Therapeutic Drug Carrier Systems*. This is essential not only for all pharmacy collections but for those in biomedical engineering and even for some collections in surgery. Somewhat less "mechanical" but of similar mission is Elsevier's *Advanced Drug Delivery Reviews*. Many of its numbers are thematic and contain two to five interrelated reviews. This title is strongly recommended for larger pharmaceutical and pharmacological collections.

For collections emphasizing the body's processing of drugs from their ingested original form through to their excreted state, Dekker's *Drug Metabolism Reviews* is worthwhile. As this is a central theme of pharmacology, most medical and graduate pharmacy schools will need this title, although it has less immediacy for chemists.

The demand for toxicology reviews has generated the rise of *Critical Reviews in Toxicology*, a softbound from CRC-Lewis Press that favors very lengthy state-of-the-art surveys. This title is somewhat more slanted to ingested poisonings, still the mainstream approach, than is Springer's hardbound triannual, *Reviews of Environmental Contamination and Toxicology.* The American title is the first choice in most clinical settings. The German title is to be preferred where environmental regulation of factory wastes, and the like, is of greater concern.

## JOURNALS FOR ORIGINAL RESEARCH IN PHARMACOLOGY AND RELATED FIELDS THAT ALSO FEATURE REVIEWS

A number of pharmacology journals primarily intended for original research feature valuable reviews on an occasional basis. Sorting them out is best done by type of review and nationality of publisher.

Some of the more prominent titles stress minireviews. Plenum's *Pharmaceutical Research*, the *Journal of Pharmaceutical Sciences* from the American Pharmaceutical Association, and the *Journal of Medicinal Chemistry* from the American Chemical Society, are U.S. leaders in minireviews. *General Pharmacology,* and *Comparative Biochemistry and Physiology, Section C, Comparative Pharmacology* (two modestly ranking titles) and *Biochemical Pharmacology* (a leader) from Pergamon frequently present minireviews, often from British or Commonwealth authors. The *European Journal of Clinical Pharmacology*, a Springer title and German leader, and *Pharmacology and Toxicology* from Munksgaard, a Scandinanvian counterpart, are among the minireview sources on the Continent. Canadians have a regular series of brief life-and-times reviews such as the "Merck Frosst Awards" in their *Canadian Journal of Physiology and Pharmacology*. Short, tutorial reviews, termed "Primers," are frequent in the *American Journal of Hospital Pharmacy*.

However, there are still some pharmacology journals that feature occasional longer state-of-the-art reviews, including prominent American series such as "Therapeutic Reviews and Perspectives" within Lippincott's *Journal of Clinical Pharmacology*, and "Current Trends Reviews" in Wiley's *Drug Development Research*. Reviews in the *Journal of Natural Products*, from the American Society for Pharmacognoscy are second in importance only to those in *Natural Products Reports*.

Leading U.K. sources include Blackwell's *British Journal of Clinical Pharmacology*, and Academic's *Pharmacological Research*.

Continental audiences will find lengthy reviews in the *European Journal of Pharmacology* from Elsevier. At first glance it would appear that by doing this Elsevier would be undercutting its own *Trends* and *Progress* series. But the reviews in the *European* are much longer than those in *Trends* and much broader than in the *Medicinal Chemistry* series. Kluwer also fields a significant Continental title with occasional reviews: *Investigational New Drugs*.

The Asian pharmacological community has been growing, and Singapore, as much as Japan, is becoming a publishing center. Reviews are frequently found in Singapore University's *Asia Pacific Journal of Pharmacology* and the Japanese Pharmacological Society's *Japanese Journal of Pharmacology*. Both Singapore and Japan still have a way to go, however, before they catch up with New Zealand's ADIS Press. Its title, *Drugs*, already has a truly international authorship, circulation and a regular supply of review papers.

Disease-specific or organ-system-specific journals also feature reviews. Among the more prominent new entries are the "State-of-the-Art Lectures" in *Cardiovascular Drugs and Therapy* from Kluwer.

Toxicology has a healthy number of review sources among its research journals, more than any other specialty in the pharmacologically related sciences. Most toxicology journals favor lengthy state-of-the-art surveys. The American leader is *Toxicology and Applied Pharmacology* which has a "Current Issues in Toxicology" review series. Its companion Society of Toxicology series, *Fundamental and Applied Toxicology*, has similar reviews, although they are generally untitled as a series. Both serials are handled for the society by Academic Press. At a somewhat lower level of urgency, one might add Dekker's *Journal of Toxicology*, which features "Toxin Reviews."

British toxicology journals also feature reviews. The three most prominent U.K. sources for full-length reviews are *Toxicon* from Pergamon, *Human and Experimental Toxicology* from Macmillan, and *Xenobiotica* from Taylor and Francis. (Xenobiotics are any substances that are introduced to the body that are normally foreign to it. While most medicines are synthetic and are therefore technically xenobiotics, a good many of the papers in *Xenobiotica* deal with frankly harmful foreign substances.)

Continental review work in toxicology is spearheaded by Elsevier's *Chemico-Biological Interactions*, which historically had a French base, and by Springer's *Archives of Toxicology*, which had a German base. Both feature largely state-of-the-art essays.

## SYMPOSIA AND THEME ISSUES IN PHARMACOLOGY AND TOXICOLOGY

Conference literature is extremely abundant in pharmacology. Symposia serve not only to inform physicians and pharmacologists but as a venue to pitch new drugs to them. Drug companies are very common underwriters of these events, and of their publication.

A number of the sources listed in the reviews section also do conferences. These include the *Canadian Journal of Physiology and Pharmacology* from that country's National Research Council, *Drugs* from ADIS (as many as five meeting supplements a year), and the *Asia Pacific Journal of Pharmacology* from Singapore U.

Other sources not particularly known for reviews feature frequent conferences. Special symposium issues are common in *Arzneimittelforschung* from Cantor, *Archiv der Pharmazie* from VCH, the *British Journal of Pharmacology*, the *Journal of Pharmacy and Pharmacology* from the Royal Pharmacological Society (U.K.), and *Agents and Actions* from Birkhauser.

While the major U.S. pharmacology organizations certainly do hold massive annual conventions–the American Society for Pharmacology and Experimental Therapeutics tends to hold theirs in conjunction with other FASEB groups and to use the *FASEB Journal*'s abstracts editions to publish the advance text of talks–full-text reproduction of conference talks is much more common in more specialized journals than within the principal American journals of general pharmacological sciences.

There are numerous examples of more specialized conference literature. Medicinal chemists are often encountered in symposia issues of *Chirality* (a Wiley journal focusing on three-dimensional rearrangments of organic substances). Conferences on drugs to fight infectious diseases are featured in the *Journal of Antimicrobial Therapy* from Academic. Heart disease drugs are the topics of conventions reported in the *Journal of Cardiovascular Pharmacology* from Raven Press, and *Cardiovascular Drugs and Therapy* from Kluwer. Selected papers are reproduced in full text from symposia appropriate to the audience of Pergamon's *International Journal of Immunopharmacology*. The conference literature of cancer chemotherapy is covered in literally dozens of journals of oncology and hematology, with pharmacologists increasingly inclined to turn to symposia in *Anti-Cancer Drug Design* from Oxford.

As drugs get closer to the market stage, the pattern of using more special pharmacology journals for sponsored symposia often switches to using specialty medical journals for symposia. The idea is that the physicians in that specialty will be more likely to actually prescribe the medicine once they see it discussed in their own journals. Further, pharmaceutical firms know that larger pharmacology collections will take at least the leading journals of internal medicine. (See the chapter on journals of physiology and related areas of internal medicine.)

Yet another tack to covering the main findings of conferences is found in both Elsevier's *Trends in the Pharmacological Sciences* and in Plenum's *Pharmaceutical Research*. They offer conference highlight stories. These are not summaries of all the individual talks, so much as good technical reportage of the principal points and themes of the conference. The poisons segment of the profession uses this approach in the "Symposium Overview" series within *Fundamental and Applied Toxicology* from Academic.

## METHODS AND RULES IN THE PHARMACOLOGICAL AND TOXICOLOGICAL SCIENCES

It has long been a truism that most of what goes into a person is covered by one regulatory agency or another, and this is becoming the case with much of the input of man into the environment as well. Whether or not these agencies do their jobs and are right or practical in their decisions is a matter of politics. What is clear to librarians is that an enormous amount of methods literature in pharmacology and toxicology is tied up with permissible limits of contaminants or with minimum effective dosages and the like. Most libraries that have anything to do with the drug industry will have substantial literature concerning proper procedure and standards.

The leading official publication for drug makers is the *Pharmacopeial Forum* from the U.S. Pharmacopeia, a voluntary but expert organization devoted to the highest standards of professional practice in drug manufacturing and dispensing. It contains many advisories and position papers, but also features some research reviews, and theme and symposia issues. It is absolutely essential in all pharmaceutical libraries and in most large clinical collections. Having less official sanction and dealing at least partly with the commercial and engineering aspects of large drug manufacturing operations is Dekker's *Drug Development and Industrial Pharmacy*. Like the *Forum*, however, it features reviews and special theme issues.

Drug manufacturing libraries and most schools of pharmacy should also have two journals devoted to the most common "new" (1970s) technology for drug delivery. These are the *Journal of Microencapsulation* from Taylor and Francis, and the *Journal of Controlled Release* from Elsevier. Both titles stress the use of various waxy, fatty, membranous, or microcellular coatings on tiny beads that go into pills, capsules, or even transdermal patches in such a way that given medicines slowly dissolve into the body at a measured rate.

The leading methods title for the calculation of the rate of a drug's spread through the body is Plenum's *Journal of Pharmacokinetics and Biopharmaceuticals*. Pharmacokinetics is intimately tied to the judgement of how often a given medicine must be administered and goes to the heart of issues of how it might be routed (orally, intravenously, intramuscularly, etc.). Wiley has a solid competitor in this field that is also strongly recommended: *Biopharmaceutics and Drug Disposition*. It has a somewhat more British tone to it than the Plenum entry, and makes an excellent complement to the largely American authorship in the first title. ADIS offers a third choice: *Clinical Pharmacokinetics*. As is seen with other ADIS titles, there is a truly widespread base of authorship, including excellent U.S. laboratory representation.

While most drug trials on humans are the domain of licensed

physicians and are reported in journals of internal medicine, pharmacologists have some pertinent literature. Elsevier, for example features the *Journal of Clinical Research and Pharmacoepidemiology*; Raven supports *Therapeutic Drug Monitoring.* Both journals are necessary to any hospital collection that is regularly a part of clinical trials. All drug companies have to keep track of "ADR's"–adverse drug reactions–and this literature supports that activity closely. Continued approval of drugs is conditioned on the manufacturer keeping track of what ill effects are likely to occur millions of doses after initial release. (To a lesser degree, most of the journals mentioned in previous sections of this chapter with the word "clinical" involve trials work.)

It should be noted that there are many technical notes of a practical, generally chemical nature in most journals of pharmacy. The *Journal of Pharmaceuticals Sciences* from the American Pharmaceutical Association and *Pharmaceutical Research* from Plenum are probably the two leaders in this regard. The "wet chemistry" in these labs is nowadays often preceded by computer chemistry: theoretical studies of the surface of the microbe or diseased cell, and of the drug molecule that will destroy or modify the target. More and more medicinal chemists are computer modelling the interactions in terms of "docking" or "receptor" sites on the target, and calculating which conformations (3-dimensional shapes) allow for the deepest penetration or most lasting dwell time. This molecular efficiency is important to calculating how much of a medicine is needed. It also helps the pharmaceutical firm decide which chemicals are likely to be so ineffective as to be unlikely to be worth testing in the first place, and can help pinpoint problems with toxic side-effects. A major stress in pharmacology today involves reducing the number of compounds that are actually tried so as to limit expensive and sometimes controversial animal testing. (Pergamon's *Toxicology In Vitro*, and Princeton Science's *Cell Biology and Toxicology* are representative of titles that use cell cultures from humans or animals as a substitute for tests on live animals that will later have to be destroyed. Certain traditional journals of cell biology such as the *Journal of Cellular Physiology* from Wiley, the *American Journal of Physiology: Cell Physiology* from the American Physiological Society, and *In Vitro* from the Tissue Culture

Association, have thrived owing to more fundamental research involving cell lines that also do not require repeated destruction of large numbers of animals. While direct testing of drugs is not always the case in these journals, one can see that much of the effort is funded for the long term interests of pharmacology.

The major journals reporting theoretical and design studies include a first choice: *Quantitative Structure-Activity Relationships* from VCH, and a pair of second choices: the *Journal of Molecular Graphics* from Butterworth and the *Journal of Computer-Aided Molecular Design* from ESCOM Science Publishers. A number of related journals have somewhat less emphasis on drug design problems but include useful technical information for either computer graphics or related biomedical computing problems. These include the *Journal of Chemical Information and Computer Sciences* from the American Chemical Society, *Computer Methods and Programs in Biomedicine* from Elsevier, and *Computer Applications in the Biosciences* from IRL Press.

Some of the significant journals covering conventional general purpose testing for toxicology include Wiley's *Journal of Applied Toxicology*, Raven's *Toxicology Methods*, and Elsevier's *Journal of Pharmacological and Toxicological Methods*. Two journals that stress toxicological analysis of other ingested products are *Food Additives and Contaminants* from Hemisphere, and *Food and Chemical Toxicology* from Pergamon. Given the fact that many toxicology centers do contract work not only for the food but for the cosmetics and over-the-counter drug industries, these are highly worthwhile titles. Despite its more encompassing title, *Veterinary and Human Toxicology* from Kansas State University is overwhelmingly concerned with livestock as opposed to its farmers or meat products consumers, and is a primary title mostly for animal science and agriculture collections.

Most toxicology collections will need some analytical chemistry journals for detection and measurement. Unlike the core toxicology titles, these do not dwell as much on the mechanism by which the poison damages the subject, so much as how one might find whether or not a given toxin or therapeutic medicine was present in the first place.

The *Journal of Pharmaceutical and Biomedical Analysis* is

aimed both towards the detection of the relatively normal break-down of drugs within the body and the less desirable breakdown within stored pharmaceutical products. Some of the papers address the normal metabolism of therapeutic drugs after ingestion, but many are concerned with drug quality control during the manufacturing process or on the shelf. Likewise, *Clinical Chemistry,* from the American Association for Clinical Chemistry, is concerned with a broad range of medical tests, and includes the measurement of blood or urine levels of given drugs or poisons. The *Journal of Analytical Toxicology* from Preston is specifically designed to detect known poisons. While the scope of *Forensic Science* from the American Academy of Forensic Scientists includes a broad scope of topics including accident investigation and determination of the age of corpses and the like, a substantial amount of information on determining overdoses of therapeutic drugs or the presence of illegal drugs is often offered. The *Journal of the Association of Official Analytical Chemists* focuses on food and agricultural products, and is important because this society has a certain "certification" status. *Inhalation Toxicology* from Hemisphere covers airborne contaminants and contains more biological studies than most detection-oriented titles.

Few fields are as fraught with safety and liability concerns as pharmacology and toxicology. Not only are there concerns with how patients and victims will fare after ingesting these substances but there is substantial concern for inadvertant exposure of toxics in the chemical workers who make and package the drugs. Two journals emphasize lengthy reviews and policy statements that have particular importance for the handling and disposal of these materials and their byproducts in the light of the law and the consensus of the best available technology. These are Academic's *Regulatory Toxicology and Pharmacology* and Hemisphere's *Toxic Substances Journal.* The first is more focused on the drug industry in particular; the second provides a good interface of the drug industry with other chemical and industrial providers of potential pollution and poisonings.

# Genes and Development,
# Normal and Abnormal

Much to the surprise of many observers, genetics has not become entirely a mere subset of biochemistry and molecular biology. Genetics got its start with the observation of inherited traits and the quest for understanding of both superior development in agriculture and multigenerational illness in medicine. It is the geneticist's balancing of an emphasis on demonstrable, often life-effecting traits (technically called "phenotypes") along with an emphasis on the chromosomes themselves that makes genetics directionally different from approaches that look to the nucleotide linkages within genes first and later on to visible traits. In analyzing the commute we call the life of an individual, molecular biologists tend to study the auto parts to predict the arrival at the destination, while geneticists work backward from destinations and explain breakdowns and detours after the fact.

Geneticists are interested in three major themes. These are the statistical occurence of normal and abnormal traits, the environmental exposures (usually chemical or ionizing radiation) that alter normal traits, and changes in traits in large populations over long periods of time (the geneticist's contribution to evolutionary theory). For geneticists, statistics are a key early warning tool that starts the subsequent search for specific sites of molecular alteration, such as a chromosome break or mutant sequence. This "evidence of meaningful differences approach" gives gene mappers in fields as diverse as clinical genetics and extinction theory a sense of

[Haworth co-indexing entry note]: "Genes and Development, Normal and Abnormal." Stankus, Tony. Co-published simultaneously in The Serials Librarian (The Haworth Press, Inc.) Vol. 27, No. 2/3, 1995, pp. 103-112; and: Special Format Serials and Issues: Annual Review of . . . , Advances in . . . , Symposia on . . . , Methods in . . . (ed: Tony Stankus) The Haworth Press, Inc., 1995, pp. 103-112. Single or multiple copies of this article are available from The Haworth Document Delivery Service [1-800-342-9678, 9:00 a.m. - 5:00 p.m. (EST)].

*103*

direction that is badly needed in organisms like man that may have as many as three billion starting points among his chromosomes. That is not to say that the total sequencing of all of man's chromosomes, the ongoing Human Genome Project, will not one day be done. It is just more likely that areas that are involved in defects or disease will be mapped sooner.

Developmental biology is a much older field than genetics. Yet the two fields work hand in hand today. Historically the developmentalist sketched the growth of embryos of advanced animals or mapped the metamorphosis of insects. Today, the developmentalist analyzes all kinds of transformations involving simple cells that later diversify into more functional tissues with a wide variety of specialized cells–a process called differentiation. In the latter part of this century, developmental biology has also acknowledged that the nucleic acids that make up genes are the fundamental determinatives of such developments, and have therefore immersed themselves in studies of chromosome structure and function much like the geneticists. Developmentalists see genes much like the same set of directions given, one at a time, to many individual kids headed for identical destinations. But developmental biologists have been watching kids for a long time before nucleic acids were known. They have at least two centuries of observing the anatomical formations and malformations of embryonic kids under the microscope. The developmentalists see that despite the fundamental sameness of the directions given to each kid, the trip that actually results can nonetheless result in different paths to the same destination, different times of arrival at that destination, and even unintended ultimate destinations. Developmentalists today argue that not only are genetic mishaps at fault, but so are larger processes of multicellular physiology, prenatal nutrition, problems of insufficient anatomical support, and physical injury. These factors might be analogous in the story of the kid's trip to the effects of traffic, different lunchboxes, the condition of the sidewalk, and even the weather. Even when the trip ends successfully, developmentalists continue to ask themselves just how the kids prenatally "know" the intricate timing of stops and directional turns that occur on the road to differentiation, when it is not at all clear from those two hundred years of observation that genes or kids, always pay attention to the map they have. Developmentalists seek to understand just what kinds of events influence what strict molecular biologists might claim to be an exquisitely pre-planned sequence. Developmentalists have also brought along a wide number of experimental animals on which to test both genetic and environmental hypotheses.

Working together, geneticists and developmentalists are chroniclers of passages in early lifetimes that still remain in many respects, uncertain of result, and surprising in their variety of outcomes. Developmentalists represent another class of early warning scouts for geneticists, for they are the initial examiners of abnormally developed organisms (teratogenies) or those that grow at unexpected or erratic rates. Developmentalists often make the first call as to whether or not the unfortunate phenomenon is the result of a mishap on the macroscale (fetal environment) or is a matter for chromosome probing. Furthermore, while strict interpretations of cancers as resulting from misguided embryonic tissues are on the decline, developmentalists offer geneticists tremendous insights into how a single cell with damaged chromosomes can develop into the masses of cells we call tumors.

In a separate alliance, evolutionary geneticists also come together with ecologists, anthropologists, and population biologists to see just how genes and traits affect the survival of the organisms that house them: asking in effect, how the genes save themselves from extinction. Moreover, by observing similarities in gene sequences or gene-influenced biochemsitry, evolutionary geneticists are redrawing the family trees of man and animals against theories based on similarities in embryonic development or adult anatomical features.

## REVIEWS IN GENETICS AND DEVELOPMENT IN MULTISCIENCE JOURNALS AND IN SERIALS DEVOTED PRIMARILY TO REVIEWS

Genetics and development seem to merit reviews in the major multiscience journals largely when the gene for some disease is finally located or when extinction or unwanted hybridization threatens the genome of some rare plant or animal. While both clinical and evolutionary genetics collections should be certain to have *Science* and *Nature*, the former will also need *BioEssays*, *Cell* and the *FASEB Journal*, while the latter is very likely to need the *American Naturalist* and *Evolution* as alternatives. Developmentalists will do well enough following the review hunting paths of their clinical genetics counterparts.

The genetics community has a fairly compact assortment of "must-buy" review serials. The *Annual Review of Genetics* from the not-for-profit Annual Reviews, Inc. is an affordable choice for all libraries. The second choice also seemed just as clear until recently: Elsevier's *Trends in Genetics*. Many of its minireviews have a tutorial bent, making it quite suitable for many undergraduate collections. It also covers topics in differentiation to a much greater degree than the *Annual Review*, making it highly appealing to developmentalists. *Trends* sometimes comes with a "scientific centerfold" suitable for posting in instructional labs for visual clarification of a complex topic. Its relatively steep price was its only drawback, and that seemed tolerable, given that no other general genetics review was really in contention as a second choice, particularly in small or medium sized collections. But a new entry, to be mentioned in the development section, may challenge *Trends*.

Most genetics collections at large institutions that have a strong molecular biology program will also need *Mutation Research–Reviews in Genetic Toxicology*, another Elsevier entry. Here the stress is on chemical, radiational, dietary, or other environmental factors that induce chromosome breakage or that otherwise alter chromosomes at specific sites. Most of its essays feature a lengthy state-of-the-art format. The cost of this Elsevier entry is steep but the interest in this area is so strong that many research collections in public or occupational health will need it in addition to its usual subscribers at doctoral level programs in universities and in major medical schools.

The developmental community has one important hardbound series, *Current Topics in Developmental Biology*, from Academic. While in the past it has played an important role as a somewhat irregular thematic hardbound, it has more recently decided to convert to a format with essays on a variety of topics issued on a highly reliable yearly schedule. In many respects, this is a wise move. There is no competing with *Annual Review*, and the competition in the theme-symposia genre is heating up.

*Current Topics* had long faced some rather capable direct competition in the theme-symposia arena from a recurring special supplement to a regular journal, *Development*, of the (British) Company of Biologists, a title which which will be discussed later. But now an aggressive new American entry from Current Science publishers, *Current Opinion in Genetics and Development,* has entered the fray. This contender is "coincidentally" priced about the same as its *Trends in Genetics* competition. It has a format that features a theme for each issue, with each paper essentially a minireview of some subset of that theme. What is particularly intriguing about these minireviews is the frankness of the author's criticism of others' works and the author's "weighted bibliographies" that follow the minireviews. (Papers are given one or two "bullseye" marks for being particularly good, in a manner similar to movie or restaurant guides!) The merging of the topics of genetics and development place it squarely in the path of the *Trends* series. At this early stage of the competition, it seems as if *Current Opinion* might be a better choice than *Trends* for a more sophisticated audience. *Trends*, however, still leads in collections with some beginners among the readership.

## REVIEWS IN GENES AND DEVELOPMENT IN JOURNALS DEVOTED PRIMARILY TO REPORTING ORIGINAL RESEARCH

Most genetics journals publish reviews only on an intermittent basis. Delightfully, one of the two leaders, *Genetics* from the Genetics Society of America, regularly features "Perspectives." These are life-and-times minireviews, often done by major figures in their retiring years and containing autobiographical insights. *Molecular and General Genetics* from Springer, the strongest competitor of *Genetics,* is more typical. It intermittently publishes minireviews and these deal with more current matters. Lesser general genetics journals like *Hereditas* from the Scandinavian Association of Geneticists, *Somatic Cell and Molecular Genetics* from Plenum, and *Chromosoma* from Springer all publish fairly lengthy, but infrequent, reviews. The *Journal of Heredity,* now an Oxford University Press title but still having a long history in largely American agricultural genetics, tends to feature reviews on an irregular basis, although a fair number of them involve a life-and-times format, not unlike those seen in *Genetics*.

Journals dealing with medical genetics are much more fervent in producing reviews. The *American Journal of Human Genetics*, a Chicago title, has at least three categories: "Review," "Invited Review," and "Hypothesis." *Human Genetics* from Springer tends to have somewhat fewer reviews than *AJHG*, but still many more than *Molecular and General Genetics*, its aforementioned partner for nonclinical work. Wiley's *Genetic Epidemiology* is typical of many clinical titles with its stress on regular editorial minireviews.

Cancer genetics is a tremendously booming area with many articles or original research in need of some kind of corraling by review. Frequent, fairly short editorial reviews tend to dominate in Macmillan's *Oncogene*, in Elsevier's *Cancer Genetics and Cytogenetics*, in Wiley's *Genes, Chromosomes, and Cancer*, and in IRL's *Carcinogenesis*. Most cancer genetics collections will also need certain of the more fundamental research journals in oncology for their reviews from major research centers. This is particularly the case with reviews in the *Journal of the National Cancer Institute*, and *Cancer Research* from the American Association for Cancer Research, two titles that bridge clinical and fundamental work. A new title from the latter group, *Cancer Epidemiology, Biomarkers, and Prevention*, is announcing a full range of regular reviews, invited minireviews, and editorial reviews. These will bring together perspectives on the statistical occurrence of cancers, their salient molecular dislocations, and environmental factors that might be eliminated in order to reduce the chromosomal damage that leads to the cancers in the first place.

The idea of inserting new genes into human chromosomes after amplifying "good" genes through PCR (polymerase chain reaction) techniques is relatively new but its leading journal, *Human Gene Therapy*, from Mary Anne Liebert, has also a policy of regular editorial minireviews.

General developmental biology has many fewer reviews than genetics, although work relating to the development of cancers is clearly increasing. The leading journals, *Developmental Biology* from Academic, and *Genes and Development* from Cold Spring

Harbor, almost never feature reviews. "Essays in Development," largely state-of-the-art reviews, is a valuable but an infrequent item in *Development*, a journal from the (British) Company of Biologists. More encouragingly, *Roux's Archives of Developmental Biology* from Springer has begun a "Landmarks in Developental Biology" series that parallels the "Perspectives" series of *Genetics* in its life-and-times tone. Given the much longer history of developmental biology, few of the papers are autobiographical. *Developmental Genetics* from Wiley has infrequent state-of-the-art papers.

Certain traditional journals of embryology and microscopic anatomy, particularly Karger's *Anatomy and Embryology* and Wiley's *Developmental Dynamics* feature exceptionally lengthy papers of normal development. Many of them contain extensive literature reviews. Abnormal development is explored in similarly lengthy papers in Wiley's *Teratology* and in its *Teratogenesis, Carcinogenesis, and Mutagenesis*. Briefer "Research Capsules" are increasingly common in *Cell Growth and Differentiation* from the American Association for Cancer Research. This journal is clearly a rising star and has more general relevance for developmentalists than its cancer affiliation alone suggests.

## SYMPOSIA AND THEME ISSUES IN GENES AND DEVELOPMENT

While general geneticists meet regularly and have an annual abstracts issue of *Genetics* to show for it, the specialists in human genetics are much more gregarious and prolific. All three of the major clinical journals, the *American Journal of Human Genetics* from Chicago, the *American Journal of Clinical Genetics* from Wiley, and *Human Genetics* from Springer, regularly feature symposia and theme issues. Even those titles not specifically devoted to cancer epidemiology like Wiley's *Genetic Epidemiology* and Karger's *Cell Genetics and Cytogenetics* are highly active in symposia and theme issue publishing.

Recombinant DNA workers in Europe will definitely need the symposia in Elsevier's *Gene*, for congresses related to advances in manipulative technique leading to the introduction of favorable genes, usually into industrial microbes rather than into humans.

Researchers in mutation research are given an annual convention abstracts issue with a subscription to Wiley's *Environmental and Molecular Mutagenesis.* It covers the meetings of the U.S.-based Environmental Mutagen Society, while *Mutagenesis* from the IRL/ Oxford University Press handles abstracts for the proceedings of the U.K. Environmental Mutagen Society. Full-text symposia talks of the European Environmental Mutagen Society are becoming a frequent feature of Elsevier's *Mutation Research.*

Arguably the most important series for many molecularly-inclined geneticists is the *Cold Spring Harbor Symposia on Quantitative Biology,* from Cold Spring Harbor Press. This annual "live" summer conference is held at the world famous research center and summer retreat on Long Island, a place run by Nobel Laureate James Watson of DNA fame. Not only is the full text of many of the presentations provided, but several pages of candid photos of the many distinguished participants are featured. (Nobel Prizewinners look just as silly as the rest of us in resort wear.)

The evolutionary segment of human genetics is covered in part in the *Yearbook of Physical Anthropology* (a supplement to Wiley's *American Journal of Physical Anthropology*) and by occasional symposia in *Human Biology* from Wayne State University Press.

Developmentalists in the U.S. tend not to have their own convention and symposia publications. Some of their best presentations tend to appear in the symposia outlets of neighboring disciplines. They tend to have a fair number of full-text papers in the *Annals of the New York Academy of Sciences,* a nominally multiscience thematic series with a *de-facto* preponderance of life science papers. Abstracts from developmentalists are also frequent in the annual convention issue of the American Society of Cell Biology, a supplement to the *Journal of Cell Biology.* Developmentalists whose interest is primarily evolutionary will more occasionally have the full text of major talks of symposia in their fields covered in the *American Zoologist,* the theme-issue journal of the American Society of Zoologists. Arguably the strongest and by far the most regular source of symposia publications in developmental biology are the thematic supplements to *Development,* the Company of Biologists journal. In these, the full text of talks given at topically focused meetings of the British Society for Developmental Biology are presented. These supplements are, like the journal, hardbound and excellently illustrated. If *Development* is for some reason not already in the collection, extra effort to obtain these volumes through separate purchase ought to be made.

## SERIAL SOURCES OF METHODS IN GENETICS AND DEVELOPMENT

Useful reference data papers are common in many journals of genetics, as the means of sequencing normal and mutant chromosomes, and the creation of copies of those sequences, multiply. The 1980s saw an explosion of mutation methods papers; the 1990s will see a massive stress on building libraries of standardized sequences. The study of genes (and the proteins for which they encode) within an evolutionary context has experienced a slower, but steadier growth. The following are listed in a geographic sequence. First we will treat Continental European sources, then British and former Commonwealth sources, and then finally, American sources. Ironically, with one or two exceptions, the more expensive sources that are listed first are not as valuable as their less expensive American counterparts.

No less than four Elsevier publications have methods and data papers in abundance. They effectively cover much of the Continental European effort along these lines. These include the aforementioned *Trends in Genetics* ("Technical Tips"), *Gene* (many "Short Communications" are methods notes), and *Mutation Research* (a whole subseries on "Genetic Toxicology Testing"). The fourth Elsevier title is virtually all methods papers: *Gene Analysis Techniques*. Springer's principal entry in the mutation research area is *Radiation and Environmental Biophysics*, a title which, while not solely devoted to x-ray chromosomal damage, focuses on this area. The *Journal of Molecular Evolution* from Springer has the highest standing among all of these Continental titles respective to its field.

British efforts have focused on sections in three publications. There are the "Database Papers" of known mutant sequences within *Mutagenesis*, a special section, entitled "DNA Damage," within Taylor and Francis's longstanding *International Journal of Radiation Biology*, and a new title from the British branch of Wiley,

*Disease Markers*, which is almost wholly given over to the biochemical markers of illnesses that are inherited or the result of environmentally mutated genes.

U.S. efforts are well represented by exhaustive survey papers published in special supplements to *Environmental and Molecular Mutagenesis*. These typically detail the results of dozens of new chemical agents tested on experimental animals or microorganisms for chromosome breakage. *Radiation Research* from Academic has a substantial number of papers on x-ray induced damage. *Biochemical Genetics* from Plenum is a journal of moderate rank in both the medical genetics and evolutionary genetics communities. *Molecular Biology and Evolution* from the University of Chicago is clearly one of the leaders, sharing the top with *American Naturalist* and those evolutionary papers in *Genetics*. Only the *Journal of Molecular Evolution* from Springer comes close.

Developmental biology has been seeing fewer and fewer methods papers and no new dedicated journals in methodology. Gross anatomical observations and surgical methods of normal embryo manipulation have long reached the handbook stage. The literature of teratological inductions on the microscopic level has been taken over by pharmacologists and toxicologists who work with enormous batches of embryos when screening for birth defects potentials during drug trials. One of the more important exceptions has been the collaborative work of developmentalists, geneticists, pathologists, and surgeons in the *Journal of Craniofacial Genetics and Developmental Biology* from Munksgaard.

# Infection, Immunity, Allergy, and Autoimmunity

Even after it was discovered that microbes caused infectious diseases, at least two important questions were posed for each disease. The first asked what particular microbe caused a particular disease. The second asked why only some of those people exposed to that microbe caught the disease full force, while others either had it mildly or resisted it altogether. The answers to this second question were to eventually open up explanations for diseases that were long known not to be infectious at all.

The medical history of the 19th and early 20th centuries was dominated by the announcements of new causative microbes found for various infections. The bacterially-based specialties of infectious diseases and epidemiology were strongly on the ascendant. In many cases, diseases within their domain were beaten back with the improved preservation of food, or the public health approach of greater cleanliness, and isolation or removal of sources of infection. Certain new drugs called antibiotics and antiseptics were developed that killed many bacteria outright. These drugs were generally the result of the cooperation of the infectious disease specialists and pharmaceutical firms, an alliance that remains important today.

With time, the development of vaccines as either preventative or cure came to the fore, and for a while this approach also remained predominantly within the realm of infectious disease specialists. Early approaches to vaccine making recapitulated early philosophical theories of "whole body" or "sound body" immunity to dis-

[Haworth co-indexing entry note]: "Infection, Immunity, Allergy, and Autoimmunity." Stankus, Tony. Co-published simultaneously in *The Serials Librarian* (The Haworth Press, Inc.) Vol. 27, No. 2/3, 1995, pp. 113-126; and: *Special Format Serials and Issues: Annual Review of . . . , Advances in . . . , Symposia on . . . , Methods in . . .* (ed: Tony Stankus) The Haworth Press, Inc., 1995, pp. 113-126. Single or multiple copies of this article are available from The Haworth Document Delivery Service [1-800-342-9678, 9:00 a.m. - 5:00 p.m. (EST)].

*113*

ease. The notion of infectious disease episodes was anthropomorphi- sized into a sometimes moralistic melodrama of a "strong constitution" versus a "weak constitution," with cowardly, but wildly wriggling and multiplying microbes playing the part of vil- lain, and virtuous mankind playing the part of hero. Some vaccines were made up of "constitutionally weakened" bacteria or para- sites–usually cultivated in some unsuspecting guinea pig, cow, or horse–with the extracted microbe then having been either mildly poisoned with small doses of antiseptic, or a debilitating heat steril- ization. The reduced culture was then injected into the human pa- tient. The idea was that a reasonably sound body or strong human constitution–preferrably one not itself weakened by drunkeness, impiety, sloth, constipation, or sexual vices–ought to be able to triumph over the weakened bacteria.

Early microscopes would often show a veritable battle as certain white blood cells would literally attack and eat up the prolific but unworthy bacteria. (These blood cells were called "phagocytes" from the Greek verb for eating.) There was some notion, not entire- ly incorrect, that the body would view this as a kind of athletic or military training experience and become more fit to resist later attacks by unweakened bacteria. Proof that a battle was taking place was found in the presence of a short fever (one that was hopefully milder than that of the virulent disease) or in a tolerable inflamma- tion at the site of the injection. If the vaccine caused the patient to get too sick, or subsequently failed to protect the patient against the disease, it often allowed the infectious disease specialist to assign the blame to the bad habits of the patient, as much as to a failure of medical knowledge.

Two technical developments began to undercut this moralistic scenario.

First, it became apparent that many successful vaccines did not have to contain intact bacteria. It was fortuitously discovered that even seemingly trivial fragments of dried-up cultures could be re- constituted with water, saline, or alcohol, and sometimes confer immunity after injection. Sometimes white blood cells other than the phagocytes seemed to respond to these injections and did not seem to work through an obvious gobbling of the fragments. This brought on the question: If the bogey man of the bacterium need not be present in any obvious way to bring on the virtuous counterattack, was the virtue of the patient all that important in understanding immunity? The answer, more often than not, was no, although certain behaviors and environmental factors were definitely implicated in increasing one's chances of getting some diseases, validating a continuing interest in epidemiology and public health.

The second question was related to the bacterial fragments themselves: just what sort of debris was it that conferred immunity through such small quantitites? The rise of analytical biochemistry on the microscale—amounts in milligrams—allowed the infectious disease specialist to determine what substances seemed to assist the body's immune process. Carbohydrates and fats from the bacterium, or from the blood of an animal exposed to the bacterium, sometimes stimulated an effective immune response. Much more commonly, however, proteins and fragments of nucleic acids from the bacterium, or from the blood of the exposed animal, were most effective. Some tiny granules which were to become known as antibodies seemed to represent a whole new line of the body's defense.

This view gained strength as viruses and anti-viral vaccines became better understood, because viruses are generally made up only of proteins and nucleic acids. Any immunity that these viruses triggered had to come from reactions to foreign, invading proteins or nucleic acids. A new class of medical specialists strongly grounded in the biochemistry of the immune reaction arose. They became known as immunologists. The infectious disease specialist remained, identifying the symptoms and causative microbes, and planning treatments with antibiotics. The immunologists took matters down to the molecular level and looked for the specific triggers of the inflammation reaction and the portions of the drugs or fractions of human blood or antibodies that seemed to fight the infection. It was also rather tardily discovered that the hitherto obscure thymus, a gland that actually tends to shrink in adult life, was important to immune function. It turned out that the seemingly insignificant substance we call bone marrow was not just bone cavity filler, but an important breeding ground for blood cell immune warriors. The lymph system was understood to be more than a simple drainage system. All of this anatomy and portions of other organ regions were added to immunology's domain over time, although immunologists had to share them with other specialties, particularly hematology.

An ironic breakthrough occurred when similarities between the body's immune response to infection and its response to allergenic substances became apparent on the microscale level. In double-blind studies of vaccines in which some "pseudo-vaccines" actually contained no weakened bacterial or virus fragments, some of the same fever or inflammation reactions were nonetheless observed. The reaction was to the proteins of the experimental animal that were injected. Some of the injected people simply turned out to be allergic to those proteins. And while it was observed that vaccines with no microbial components whatsoever did not confer subsequent immunity, it was also seen that both proteins from invading microbes and proteins from allergens seem to be attacked in a similar manner by the body's defenses. Some allergy treatments emphasized an innoculation style program of gradually increasing doses of the allergen so as to strengthen the body's ability to handle unprogrammed allergic exposure without so severe a reaction. Better understanding of severe reactions was particularly important for blood transfusion work. While chemical tests to sort out blood types were actually quite old, the underlying basis of the immune reaction was soon to be seen as reactions to the surface proteins of the transfused blood cells.

Another piece of correlating evidence for the links between immunity and allergy was that some pharmaceuticals that relieved the inflammation of an infection were also used to relieve the inflammation and upset of allergy attacks, suggesting an underlying similarity in the body's defense to provoking foreign substances.

Soon a second wave of inflammation-cued studies occurred, and immunology once again played an unanticipated part. Biochemical analysis of inflammatory diseases like arthritis disclosed no bacteria nor any foreign allergens, yet inflammation-responding drugs such as steroids often seemed to work much in the same way against these familiar yet unclassified diseases as they did in infection and allergy. The idea that the human body as a whole might mistakenly have an immunological reaction to some of its own parts at first seemed ludicrous. But the discovery of auto-antibodies in patients with diseases such as arthritis, rheumatism, multiple sclerosis, systemic lupus, and scleroderma turned old-thinking on its head. Ironically this discovery made an awareness of immunology a scientific necessity for other clinical specialties such as rheumatology, neurology, and even endocrinology-metabolism. It has now been decisively proved that at least juvenile diabetes is the result of autoimmune attacks on key cells within the pancreas. (Some critics still think that a virus may be the trigger for the onset of those attacks, however.)

As microscopes and microsampling of blood and tissues grew ever more powerful, the granular clusters of irritating proteins and the body's defensive proteins came to be calibrated as "complement" levels. The term complement was used because close examination showed that these opposing molecules actually locked against each other's surface peaks and gaps, "completing" each other's three-dimensional puzzle, so to speak. "Complement" levels were used as a measure, independent of patient self-reporting, of just how aggravating flare-ups of autoimmune illnesses were at any given time.

Yet another boost for immunology has come from organ transplantation and implantable artificial organs. Here the studies that began with the inflammation supressing properties of steroids have advanced into a wide variety of ways of fooling the body's antibodies into inaction, or at least managing the counterattack to these foreign tissues and substances. Even more recently, hopes of stimulating antibody attacks–the opposite approach–have been a theme of experimental cancer treatments. Here the hope is to make the body recognize the essential "foreignness" of the cancer cell and attack it much as it would an invading microbe. Ironically, one way of stimulating a body's depleted defenses has been to inject suitably matched donor marrow into bone whose native marrow has been rendered impotent by disease or medical treatment side-effects.

In a way, the research has come full circle. The infectious diseases of the 18th and 19th centuries started us on the road to understanding immunity, and now our knowledge of immunity is crucial in understanding the diseases of the 1990s, particularly AIDS. AIDS is insidious in that its virus specifically attacks antibody-making white cells in such a way that all sorts of opportunistic microbes and autoimmune reactions can eventually wreak havoc on the body unchecked. AIDS has issued a call to arms to all of the involved specialties: infectious disease, epidemiology, immunology. Libraries should be ready to respond with the review, symposia, and methods sources that help coordinate the counterattack.

## SOURCES OF REVIEWS:
## GENERAL SOURCES OUTSIDE OF IMMUNOLOGY

Reviews in our target fields are increasingly welcome in the major multiscience journals. No collection serving this audience should be without the reviews in *Science, Nature*, and the *FASEB Journal*. Some of the journals of general microbiology will occasionally feature microbes of clinical importance and the inexpensive and valuable *Annual Review of Microbiology* from Annual Reviews, Inc. should be in most medium clinical collections and in all medical schools. *Advances in Virus Research* from Academic will cover the underrepresentation of viruses in general microbiology review sources for the same level of institution. Even leading sources of cell biology will carry minireviews of papers in this area, and a subscription to *Cell* from Cell Press is certainly warranted in collections of medium size. Both the *Journal of the American Medical Association* and the *New England Journal of Medicine* frequently carry reviews in immunologically related fields, and are a natural for even the smallest collections. The *Journal of Experimental Medicine* and the *Journal of Clinical Investigation* have an overwhelming interest in the field and are prime sources of extended trials papers, and likewise belong even in local hospitals. The *American Review of Respiratory Disease* does double duty: it covers both infection and allergy in reviews and carries minireviews frequently.

## REVIEWS SOURCES AIMED AT IMMUNOLOGISTS

Nonetheless, there are plenty of important reviews explicitly marketed for the clinical infection, immunity, and allergy community. There are four unambiguous, first-round choices for even the smallest collections. The first is *Clinical Microbiology Reviews* from the

American Society for Microbiology, a softbound quarterly. It best covers overviews of the responsible germs. The second is *Epidemiologic Reviews*, an annual from Johns Hopkins which generally covers multipatient outbreaks and multi-site experiences. While all kinds of illnesses are covered, infectious disease epidemiology remains paramount, and the public health community is well served. The third is the *Annual Review of Immunology* from the not-for-profit Annual Reviews, Inc. It is a worthy representative of its distinguished hardbound genre. Fourth and finally, *Clinical Reviews in Allergy* from Humana Press covers the mundane but clinically very frequent environmental bad reactions many of us experience. All four have advantages of relatively low prices and most have wonderful impact factors. Even small hospital libraries should have these titles.

The midrange of medium sized universities with some masters degrees in allied health sciences, or teaching hospitals that do not house an entire medical school collection, is more difficult. A small number of very comprehensive, enduring, state-of-the-art essays for specialists are featured in Academic's *Advances in Immunology*. The series is very well cited and costs less than a hundred dollars or so for the one or two hardbound volumes annually. It is a first choice at this intermediate level. Its chief American rivals are the well-established *Critical Reviews in Immunology* from CRC Press, and a very new and somewhat freewheeling journal of minireview commentary, *Current Opinion in Immunology* from Current Science. The first of these softbounds is roughly quarterly, the second bimonthly. Both have a preponderance of American papers. Both cost about three times what *Advances* charges. Experience favors *Critical Reviews*, but a decision on priorities is best reserved until the leading Euro-entry is also considered. That entry is the eminently readable *Immunology Today* from Elsevier. *Immunology Today* has a variety of useful events calendars and technical tips, but is chiefly renowned for its tutorial minireviews. It is particularly important that it be included in the collection if one of the major continental journals, such as VCH's *European Journal of Immunology* or Blackwell's *Immunology* and *Scandinavian Journal of Immunology,* is not already there. Despite costing an extra hundred dollars or so, it is probably a better choice for collections with some beginners or nonspecialists than either *Critical Reviews* or *Current Opinion*. When funds are tight at the intermediate level, having *Advances* for the advanced, and *Trends* for the tyros, probably makes for the best strategy.

Assuming that all the titles already discussed have been secured in the collection, the final option is a long-established, heavily laden vault of state-of-the-art reviews, that requires a vault of money to acquire it. Nonetheless, virtually every doctoral level graduate program and comprehensive medical school must have *Immunological Reviews*. It is arguably the largest provider of scholarly reviews in any one discipline. While it represents a commitment of a few thousand dollars, it also represents the best review source out of Europe after *Immunology Today*.

## INTERMITTENT REVIEWS IN JOURNALS PRIMARILY DEVOTED TO ORIGINAL RESEARCH

A number of journals carry reviews as an adjunct to their role as reporters of original research. In a number of cases, the publishers of these journals already have lengthy-review-oriented counterparts and tend towards "minireviews" in their general purpose journals. The U.S. scene is dominated by the *Journal of Clinical Microbiology* and *Infection and Immunity* from the ASM, which also publishes *Clinical Microbiology Reviews*. *Clinical Infectious Diseases* is yet another high-standing journal, from the University of Chicago, and it also has some review function. The *Journal of Allergy and Clinical Immunology* has no American Academy of Allergy counterpart for reviews but rather itself serves as an important source of both minireview and state-of-the-art reviews. All four titles belong in most hospital collections.

The British scene has two important review sources: state-of-the-art and editorial pieces are found in both Churchill-Livingstone's *Journal of Medical Microbiology*, and in Academic's *Journal of Infection*. While both have a fairly sound track record, prices tend to favor the Academic entry. *Microbial Pathogenesis*, another topically related entry from the British branch of Academic, has begun to do as well as these older titles, but costs about as much as the more expensive Churchill-Livingstone representative. It cannot yet be recommended as strongly for its review function.

The Continental review situation is predictably complicated and expensive. Well-established German, Scandinavian, and Dutch journals all vie for attention to their reviews. The German contingent is headed by *Medical Microbiology and Immunology,* a minireview source from Springer, and the *European Journal of Clinical Microbiology and Infectious Disease* from Viewig, largely favoring lengthy-state-of-the-art works. The comprehensive review, often featured in special review supplements, is exceptionally frequent in *APMIS: Acta Pathologica, Microbiologica, et Immunologica Scandinavica* from Munksgaard. *FEMS Microbiology Immunology* is the Dutch representative, and has more occasional lengthy reviews. (*FEMS Microbiological Reviews* understandably bears the brunt of *FEMS* reviewing.) To add to the confusion, Swiss-based Birkhauser is launching *Medical Microbiology Letters,* and is actively recruiting minireview authors. There is no clear-cut winner in this group, based only on review service. Impact factors also provide few sharp indicators. Price and the notion of greater multinational representation does favor the *European Journal,* although the better endowed collections will probably want the many extensive reviews in *APMIS* as well.

Assuming that the European situation is settled, one is still left in this case with some important minireviews from other parts of the world. Japan has long been among international leaders in both infectious disease and immunologial studies, and *Microbiology and Immunology* from the Center for Academic Publications is worth considering for the largest academic collections.

## SYMPOSIA AND THEME JOURNALS

It is clear that this diverse community of scholars meets frequently, and publishes the results of those meetings on a regular basis. The leading source of American symposia and meeting reports is unambiguously Chicago's *Journal of Infectious Disease* for its sector of specialists, with Appleton and Lange's *Transplantation Proceedings* a phenomenal convocation reporter in its specialty area. The *FASEB Journal* plays a major role in reporting key papers from more general immunological conventions. These three titles are of overwhelming importance and represent first round choices for U.S. collections. *Immunological Investigations* from Dekker plays a minor role in the same capacity. More comprehensive collections might wish to take it. Collections in fundamental immunological studies might be better served by Academic's *Cell Immunology* which regularly offers a "Meeting Reports" section.

The principal American theme journals are Saunders' *Infectious Disease Clinics of North America* and *Immunology and Allergy Clinics of North America*, two venerable quarterlies with strong appeal to clinicians. They are first round choices even in small hospital collections. Less prominently, the newer *Current Opinion in Immunology* from Current Science features theme issues, and should that journal thrive, these might have a comparable appeal to a more research-oriented audience. Right now, it is optional.

The British and Europeans are just as gregarious as their American counterparts, and some of the same specialty areas thrive. *Bone Marrow Transplantation* from the British house, Macmillan, has special symposium supplements. The British division of Academic also features live symposia in its *Journal of Autoimmunity*. (Auto-immunity is covered in general purpose journals in the U.S., particularly in the *Journal of Immunology* which has added the Society for Clinical Immunology to its sponsors.) Meetings of the British Allergy Society are covered in *Clinical and Experimental Allergy*, a Blackwell title.

The French predominate in Elsevier's *Research in Immunology* which publishes a good number of "Times and Trends Symposia," theme issues, and congress reporting. Recall that this publication is anchored at Paris's famous Pasteur Institute which has a similarly formatted companion that stresses infectious diseases, *Research in Microbiology*. The Swiss house Karger fields *Immunologic Research, Inflammation and Complement*, and *Thymus*, all of which have symposia issues.

Munksgaard, the Danish publisher of the massive *Immunological Reviews*, also handles *Allergy* which reports some continental European meetings. The leading German entries are the heavily thematic and largely clinical *Springer Seminars in Immunopathology*, and

*Immunobiology* from Gustav Fischer, which has a more fundamental tone.

This assortment seems bewildering and is certainly expensive. Nonetheless, in terms of serving the symposium function, the *Springer Seminars* are clearly the winners. The rest of the collection must be looked at in terms of local subject emphases. *Bone Marrow Transplantation* clearly belongs in collections that have a heavy need of *Transplantation Proceedings*. *Research in Immunology* still has a bent toward infection-based immune responses, and is a better match for collections with an infectious disease approach. The *Journal of Autoimmunity* fits best where chronic rheumatic and sometimes metabolic diseases are the main fare. *Clinical Allergy* is probably a better value for its frequency and content for working American allergy specialists that follow the *Journal of Allergy and Clinical Immunology*.

## METHODS LITERATURE IN THE FIELD

Killing germs within patients, or preventing ill effects from germs through hygiene remain very vital and very practical topics for journals. A substantial number of journals of general clinical practice or internal medicine cover antibiotic regimens routinely, and those journals are described in the chapter on physiology. The leading journals specifically focused on the antibiotics industry are *Antimicrobial Agents and Chemotherapy* from the ASM, the *Journal of Antimicrobial Agents and Chemotherapy* from the British branch of Academic, and the *Journal of Antibiotics* from the Japan Antibiotics Research Association. This assortment represents both the traditional alliance between the infectious disease and the pharmaceuticals communities, and some of the historically strongest geographic concentrations of antibiotic research. *Antiviral Research* from Elsevier adds both a greater European perspective and a sharper focus on viruses.

While many kinds of nonmicrobial diseases are handled by the *American Journal of Epidemiology* from Johns Hopkins and the *American Journal of Public Health* from the American Public Health Association, the tracking of infectious diseases and eradication measures are still frequently reported, and most larger academic collections should have these relatively inexpensive standards. Yet another bargain with a strong, but not exclusive interest on infectious disease outbreaks is *MMWR: Morbidity and Mortality Weekly Report* from the U.S. Superintendent of Documents. (A worthwhile edition with special supplements is available from the Massachusetts Medical Society, publishers of the *New England Journal of Medicine*.) It often provides the first warning of a new outbreak. Given that Americans are traveling more than ever, and that immigration from Asia, Africa, the Carribean and Latin America continues to increase, it is not out of line for major medical centers and large urban hospitals, in particular, to consider subscriptions to the *American Journal of Tropical Medicine and Hygiene*, an economical Allen Press-managed title. Collections with a bit more money might also wish the British companion, the *Transactions of the Royal Society of Tropical Medicine and Hygiene*, and a U.N. publication, the *Bulletin of the World Health Organization*.

Many hospitals will pay for an assortment of decontamination journals on microbes that have taken up residence on their wards. Many of these are of a trade or newsletter genre and are targeted to both M.D.'s and to supervisors of nurses, supplies, and maintenance. In order of increasing costs these are *Infection Control Bulletin* from Infection Control Educational Products, the *American Journal of Infection Control* from Mosby, *Infection Control and Hospital Epidemiology* from Charles Slack, and *Hospital Infection Control* from American Health Consultants. The *Journal of Hospital Infection* is from the British branch of Academic and is the most expensive of the group. The Mosby, Slack, and Academic titles represent the higher levels of sophistication in this assortment, and are recommended in roughly this priority sequence for long term library retention.

There are three journals frankly devoted to methods in fundamental immunology. The longest-established title is Elsevier's *Journal of Immunological Methods*. Its prestige, advantages, disadvantages, and place in the library scheme of things ironically make it highly reminiscent of Elsevier's competitor Munksgaard's *Immunological Reviews*. It has literally hundreds of papers a year and belongs in all major medical schools and Ph.D. programs. Its cost at approximately $2,000 annually, however, makes it a particularly grievous burden for smaller institutions. For over a dozen years, its only competition in the methods niche was Dekker's *Journal of Immunoassay*, a vehicle of admittedly more modest reputation and about 15% of the cost. At least partly for reasons of costs and a lack of a truly impressive contender, Academic Press has recently launched *ImmunoMethods* for about 5% of the cost of the *Journal of Immunological Methods*. Given that small price, and Academic's reputation in a number of companion journals, this author is recommending a gamble on *ImmunoMethods* in both larger and smaller collections. For many collections, it may be the only methods journal they can afford.

The absence of the *Journal of Immunological Methods* or the *Journal of Immunoassay* has not meant an absolute absence of useful methods papers, particularly for clinical testing. Methods papers have been a regular feature of the ASM's *Infection and Immunity*, and most of the other major journals of immunology mentioned earlier, as well as certain journals devoted to serving laboratory medicine. *Human Immunology* from Elsevier has the largest number within the immunology community proper, but *Analytical Biochemistry* from Academic and *Clinical Chemistry* from the American Association for Clinical Chemistry are also quite strong in these areas. *Tissue Antigens* from Munksgaard has long featured papers on the immune reactions and compatability of tissues, particularly those that might be transfused or transplanted. Most collections of clinical immunology and blood transfusion reaction infection control will very much need at least *Blood* from Saunders and pragmatic bulletins like *Blood Bank Week* from the American Association of Blood Banks.

Pharmaceutical firms, particularly those with advanced biotechnology in the separation, purification, and cloning of antibodies have been making substantial headway introducing immunologically based medicines. Initial findings about these new generation "drugs" appear apart from traditional antibiotic literature, however, because many of these "drugs" are intended for allergies, noninfectious autoimmune diseases, metabolic disturbances and innovative cancer treatments. The leading journals are quite expensive and while many biotech and pharmaceutical companies will take them as a matter of course, many small hospital collections will depend on journals of clinical immunology to monitor their progress on actual patients. The most traditional allergy-oriented pharmacology journal is Birkhauser's *Agents and Actions*. The newer wave of immunopharmacology journals is headed by *Immunopharmacology* from Elsevier. Following behind at a slight distance are Pergamon's *International Journal of Immunopharmacology* and Raven's *Journal of Immunotherapy*.

## THE SPECIAL CASE OF AIDS

While AIDS reviews, symposia, and accompanying clinical testing and drug trials are exceptionally welcome in many of the major journals already discussed, a body of sharply focused literature has also emerged. Unfortunately, so has a great deal of marginally valid and/or overpriced scientific literature. At this time two highly reliable journals appear to feature the bulk of important reviews and symposia alongside their regular research articles: *AIDS Research and Human Retroviruses* from Mary Ann Liebert, a relatively new but rising star in cellular and molecular biology publishing, and the *Journal of Acquired Immunodeficiency Syndromes* from Raven, an older, sound biomedical publisher with some experience in immunology publishing. Two special review services from Dekker, a publisher with a more modest citation track record, but one which also includes some immunology titles, will soon be old enough to evaluate more fully. These are *AIDS Research Reviews* and *AIDS Clinical Review*. Both annuals are also recommended provisionally for those who have already secured the two more general purpose journals.

# Inorganic Chemistry

Inorganic chemistry–for historical reasons once defined as non-carbon-compound chemistry–is a minority specialty in a field dominated by carbon-containing "organic" compounds. Yet inorganic chemistry has kept itself from becoming considered a trivial field by aggressively expanding its agenda throughout the history of science.

From the alchemy of the Dark Ages through the birth of modern chemistry during the Enlightenment, inorganic topics dominated chemistry with a practical agenda of metals, minerals, paints, clays, and strong acids and alkalis. Many atmospheric gases were added as topics in the eighteenth century, as were certain crystalline substances in the nineteenth century.

Nonetheless, the nineteenth century began the overall domination of chemistry by those working with organic compounds. This turn of events came about because it was finally discovered that many compounds related to living things, i.e., "organic" chemicals, could actually be synthesized. Many of these "organic" compounds featured carbon-to-carbon bonds that proved amenable to a wide variety of further manipulations that proved useful to the drug and dye industries. By the early twentieth century–and partly in reaction–inorganic chemistry cleverly managed to claim for its own, out of this bounty, any compound, even those containing carbon, in which a central metal atom determined the overall molecular architecture: a subspecialty called coordination chemistry. The use of the x-ray around this time by the father and son team of W. H. and W. L. Bragg as a probe for crystal structure strengthened inorganic chem-

[Haworth co-indexing entry note]: "Inorganic Chemistry." Stankus, Tony. Co-published simultaneously in *The Serials Librarian* (The Haworth Press, Inc.) Vol. 27, No. 2/3, 1995, pp. 127-132; and: *Special Format Serials and Issues: Annual Review of . . . , Advances in . . . , Symposia on . . . , Methods in . . .* (ed: Tony Stankus) The Haworth Press, Inc., 1995, pp. 127-132. Single or multiple copies of this article are available from The Haworth Document Delivery Service [1-800-342-9678, 9:00 a.m. - 5:00 p.m. (EST)].

istry, since metal atoms within inorganic compounds gave fairly clear refraction patterns. This discovery won for them the Nobel Prize and for inorganic chemistry increased fashionability. Opportunistically, many radioactive isotopes, most nuclear fuel processing, and even particle-accelerator-made elements were eventually incorporated into radiochemical inorganic chemistry in the era encompassing the two world wars and the early Cold War era.

By the 1960s any compound in which a metal atom was directly linked to a carbon atom–whether or not the metal atom determined the overall structural characteristics–came to be dominated by what are now called organometallic chemists. In the last quarter of this century, old motivations for studying coordination and organometallic compounds like their superior catalytic abilities, were joined by two new topics. These are the use of inorganic compounds in the electronics and advanced materials industry (a major theme of today's solid-state chemistry), as well as a recognition of the important role of trace elements in body fluids and tissues in what is now termed "bioinorganic" chemistry. As a practical matter, organometallics remain by far the dominant category of inorganic compound studied, and inorganic radiochemistry has been in decline. While larger biological molecules have now shown themselves amenable to x-ray diffraction, breaking inorganic chemistry's monopoly, other types of fourier-transform assisted spectroscopy which had readier applicability in organic chemistry are now proving useful for inorganic and organometallic compounds, offsetting the loss.

## REVIEWS IN GENERAL SCIENCE AND GENERAL CHEMISTRY JOURNALS

Despite a certain increased attractiveness in the 1970s and 1980s, inorganic chemistry rarely grabs much review space in nominally multiscience sources. When a review does appear in journals like *Science* or *Nature*, the tendency is less to stress straightforward chemistry, so much as enhancements in the compound's structure or functioning caused by the presence of a metal atom. Themes in these biologically-dominated sources occasionally include new formulations for superconducting materials, but more often reviews will deal with the role of a metal atom in the folding of a protein, or the activity level of some enzyme. Bioinorganic chemists in particular will need access to the reviews in major multiscience journals like those above–and perhaps to the *Annual Review of Biochemistry*–much more often than most other inorganic chemists.

By contrast, workers apart from the bioinorganics, particularly academic and industrial inorganic workers, need reviews more in the mainstream of straightforward chemistry. Inorganic chemistry takes up a small but regular share of the leading sources of reviews for the general chemistry community. About 20% of the papers in *Chemical Reviews*, and *Accounts of Chemical Research* (both from the American Chemical Society) and *Chemical Society Reviews* (from the Royal Society of Chemistry) are devoted to inorganic, coordination, or organometallic chemistry. The highest proportion of inorganic reviews among other general chemistry sources can probably be found in *Angewandte Chemie–International Edition in English*, a VCH publication that preserves the strong German tradition in the field.

## REVIEW SOURCES DEVOTED LARGELY TO INORGANIC TOPICS

The leading sources devoted solely to reviews in general inorganic/organometallic chemistry includes five irregular hardbound series, and one annual. This vast array has both American and British wings. Together they cover the major areas of the field and represent first round selections.

On the American side, two hardbounds come to us from Academic: *Advances in Inorganic Chemistry* (a title that used to append ". . . and Radiochemistry"), and *Advances in Organometallic Chemistry*. Wiley fields *Progress in Inorganic Chemistry*, an entry with more strength in bioinorganics than its title may suggest. All are in the $100-$200 annual price range and stress lengthy state-of-the-art reviews that are among the citation leaders in their specialties.

On the British side, the Royal Society of Chemistry markets *Annual Reports on the Progress of Chemistry. Section A: Inorganic Chemistry* at approximately the same price range as the American entries but with a different editorial approach. These *Reports* feature regular columns in the various subspecialties making up the field and are prototypical installment reviews. The RSC also features a number of even more specialized installment review sources which are roughly, but not always reliably, annual. These are hardbound "Specialist Periodical Reports." Of greatest interest is the *Organometallic Chemistry SPR* series. (Other *SPRs* are narrower and will will be dealt with largely in the methods section.)

The next tier of general inorganic/organometallic review selections is markedly lower in standing. This is not so much because they lack quality as that all of them are relative latecomers to a field already well-served, and most are more expensive than the established competition. A monthly, *Comments on Inorganic Chemistry* from Gordon and Breach, is perhaps the best known of this group. Not only does it provide somewhat informal reviews, some of a tutorial type, but it occasionally features theme issues, combining two functions with one pricey subscription. *Reviews in Inorganic Chemistry* from Freund is less expensive, and while less frequent—it's a quarterly—makes a special point of getting its sometimes lengthy state-of-the-art manuscripts out very quickly after their acceptance. Many, however, appear to come from somewhat lesser known authors and labs. The relative irregularity of issuance of the leading hardbound *Advances in Organometallic Chemistry* appears to have encouraged the appearance of an annual promising promptness, *Advances in Metal-Organic Chemistry* from JAI Press, a firm better known for its librarian's titles than for its chemistry. This is the latest comer to the circle, and is too new to evaluate fairly.

Certain more specialized reviews deserve mention here. Some of them are probably better choices than the second tier of more general reviews, particularly if one's institution pays special attention to these subspecialties. *Coordination Chemistry Reviews* from Elsevier encompasses all of coordination chemistry and reaches rather deeply into more general areas of organometallic chemistry as well. *Advances in Catalysis*, an Academic Press hardbound, is the leader for metal-involved reviews for both academic and commercial audiences. The solid state inorganic chemist will typically find both Pergamon's quarterly *Progress in Solid-State Chemistry* and JAI's annual *Advances in Silicon Chemistry* of value. *Progress in Crystal Growth and Characterization* from Pergamon remains a valuable addition for industrially oriented labs. Elsevier's best specialized entry is a hardbound irregular *Advances in Inorganic Biochemistry.* Dekker features a competitor along somewhat similar lines: *Metal Ions in Biological Systems,* which has a somewhat greater stress on inorganic materials unbound to protein structures but otherwise catalyzing biological reactions. These can include papers on environmentally toxic effects as well.

## THEME ISSUES AND SYMPOSIA JOURNALS

While inorganic chemistry seems very well endowed with sources specializing in reviews, serials devoted exclusively to theme issues and symposia are generally lacking. One of the most important reasons lies in the propensity for the more British and European review and general purpose inorganic journals to sponsor symposia and *festschriften* on a fairly regular basis. Not only does one find these in leading journals already mentioned, but in other general inorganic titles like Pergamon's *Polyhedron* ("Symposia-in-Print") and Gordon and Breach's *Phosphorous, Sulfur, Silicon, and Related Elements.* The massive *Journal of Organometallic Chemistry* from Elsevier not only features more papers than any other inorganic journal, but devotes whole theme issues to overviews of recent work in given categories of elements and compounds.

## METHODS LITERATURE IN INORGANIC CHEMISTRY

Serials in this section consist of three main categories: making inorganic compounds; determining their structure; and observing them in action in catalysis, solid-state electronics, or biological systems.

While the synthesis of many categories of inorganic compounds is often featured in general purpose inorganic journals, a few niche serials are also recommended. Without a doubt the leading journal specifically devoted to their laboratory creation is the hardbound series from Wiley, *Inorganic Syntheses.* While annoyingly irregular and rather slender, it gathers within its covers some of the best time-tested procedures with an increasing concern for problems of safety. (A fair number of inorganic compounds are explosively unstable or highly toxic.) A special category of newer promising materials is covered synthetically in the *Journal of Inorganic and Organometallic Polymers* from Plenum. The first title is mandatory for even small academic collections, the second has a more likely home in industrial collections.

Most crystal structure determination has been banished from the primary journals of inorganic chemistry, largely for reasons of space. Most large working groups of inorganic chemists will need access to the methods and data reported in the three sections of the volumninous *Acta Crystallographica* from Munksgaard. Given that crystallography is no longer the only form of inorganic compound structure determination, newer methods should be collected as well. The most promising new methodology for structural studies is covered in both *Electron Spin Resonance*, an annual from CRC Press, and in the Royal Society of Chemistry's *Electron Spin Resonance B: Inorganic and Bioinorganic*, an irregular that attempts an annual issuance. While both ESR serials have a review format, the latter is a better established and more inorganically focused work. It is another in the classic British installment series, "Specialist Periodical Reports." Even those facilities which do not use ESR will find the installment reviews in the companion *Spectroscopic Properties of Inorganic and Organometallic Compounds* useful as it has a broader focus, with many references ferreting out methods papers hidden in more general journals.

Largely because catalysis by inorganic compounds has become such a titanic enterprise, papers on catalytic methods are excluded from most general inorganic journals and are generally confined to chemical engineering journals. While many such journals will have some papers on the topic, the two leaders, by far, are the *Journal of Catalysis* from Academic Press, and the *Journal of Molecular Catalysis* from Elsevier. Both have price tags to match their considerable bulk.

While novel superconducting compounds can still find their way into journals of general inorganic chemistry (and for that matter into *Science* and *Nature*) most of the compounds of eventual interest to the electronics industry are first wrestled with in the *Journal of Solid-State Chemistry* from Academic Press.

While general inorganic journals are actually increasing their coverage, the leading source of detailed bioinorganic functional papers is Elsevier's voluminous *Journal of Inorganic Biochemistry*.

# Microbiology and Biotechnology

Ever since Antonie van Leeuwenhoek microscopically discovered "microbes" in the 1500s, man has alternatingly been fascinated and afraid of them. Even before scientists learned what various microbes looked like, trades people were using them in wineries, brewing, baking, cheesemaking, and folk medicines. This chapter is primarily about serials covering the fascination and utility of microbes, and less about those dealing with their ability to cause infection or provoke an immunological response. Journals that cover those topics are in a separate chapter on infection and immunity. While bacteria have had the most prominent roles in the history of microbiology, viruses and microscopic fungi (especially yeasts) are included as microbes in many of the review, thematic, and methods journals under discussion here.

It is nonetheless largely through disease-fighting and concerns about contaminated food and water that the greatest strides in the sorting out of bacteria have been accomplished. It was recognized early on that foods and beverages could be made reasonably "bacteria proof" by one or more actions or agents: refrigeration, heating, or chemical preservatives. But the best strategy depended on which specific types of bacteria were present. It became important to know just what kinds were present in order to develop an effective plan for their control. This led to the inevitable first step of most life sciences: the systematic cataloging of the life forms under microscopical observation into families of related germs. Since bacteria were often nearly transparent, microbiologists developed stains to color them for better viewing. Certain families of bacteria

[Haworth co-indexing entry note]: "Microbiology and Biotechnology." Stankus, Tony. Co-published simultaneously in *The Serials Librarian* (The Haworth Press, Inc.) Vol. 27, No. 2/3, 1995, pp. 133-142; and: *Special Format Serials and Issues: Annual Review of . . . , Advances in . . . , Symposia on . . . , Methods in . . .* (ed: Tony Stankus) The Haworth Press, Inc., 1995, pp. 133- 142. Single or multiple copies of this article are available from The Haworth Document Delivery Service [1-800-342-9678, 9:00 a.m. - 5:00 p.m. (EST)].

*133*

could be dyed in whole or in part by one stain, while others favored different tints. This seemingly simple behavior tremendously enlarged the specialty of systematic microbiology, as more and more dyes and combinations of staining treatments led to finer distinctions.

Many of these diagnostic stains also killed the bacteria, which seemed to be a good, added effect. But this left a problem whenever scientists or hygiene experts wanted to test new stains or to compare results: consistent samples of the target microbe were often lacking. Over time it was realized that it was smarter to actually cultivate some bacteria, rather than relying on trying to isolate them from rotting sources out in the field whenever needed. This proved more of a philosophical and practical problem than at first appeared. How did one deliberately sustain something that hitherto was the target for destruction? Once again laboratory scientists looked to the food industry, where it had become long-established practice to keep a favorable strain of yeast or cheese fungi at optimum conditions from batch to batch of bread or beer. Microbiologists began to ask themselves what did bacteria require by way of nutrients, space, and waste removal to stay healthy and reproduce. This preoccupation developed academically into the fields known as microbial physiology and ecology.

For a time, systematizers would discover and describe new species, and the physiologists and ecologists would try to keep them viable, if not happy. Despite the best attempts in the lab and in the food industry, however, microbial colonies that were thought to be consistent from generation to generation showed unwanted variation among some of their members. Some of these variations were seen as spontaneous. Techniques were devised for quickly isolating these mutants to preserve the intergenerational stability of the rest of the microbial colony. It was also soon realized that despite the best efforts of scientists and food technologists, contamination by, and communication with, other microbes was partly at fault. By the 1930s, owing to the microscopical keenness of Nobel Prizewinner Joshua Lederberg, it became apparent that not only would "running with the wrong contaminated bacterial crowd" generate bad bacterial habits, it would lead to (gasp) bacterial sex. (Lederberg found that while bacteria lack sex organs as such, they do send out tubes and swap chromosomes intermittently.)

The discovery that bacteria could breed sexually lit a fire in the minds of those breeding-scientists, the geneticists. The young science of genetics became involved with bacteria because thousands of generations of bacteria could be observed over relatively short time spans. Both spontaneous mutations, and those induced by sexual transfer of chromosomal material, provided interesting examples for study. Bacterial genetics became a mainstay specialty within both genetics and microbiology. The staining science of the early systematic bacteriologists came in handy and chromosomes from one partner in a sexual breeding could sometimes be distinguished from another, and visual evidence for new combinations could also be found. In many other cases, geneticists were put onto the trail of a new mutant owing to the observations of bacterial physiologists and ecologists that the colony required some new nutrient or was producing some new waste product or required some alteration in laboratory conditions. With time it was shown that certain chemicals, x-rays, ultraviolet light, and other environmental factors could induce interesting mutations in the lab for genetics studies. This led to the specialty today known as mutation research. While mutation research, based on an analysis of events that damage chromosomes, will be treated in the chapter on genetics, microbiology literature in this chapter will include a great deal of information on the normal or standard sequences of bacterial chromosomes. Without knowing the ordinary, the location of extraordinarily good or bad sequences is hard to pinpoint.

Improvements in the ability of analytical biochemistry to detect small amounts of antibiotics and medicines coincidentally disclosed that potentially useful industrial materials and even entirely new food by-products might be generated by microbes. It became understood that bacteria and yeasts could make valuable proteins, carbohydrates, and fats that were otherwise troublesome or too expensive to produce synthetically from scratch. To these laboratory insights were added the practical experiences of bulk processors like the brewing and the petrochemicals industries. This combination enabled operations to scale up from petri dishes and test tubes to giant vats and assembly-line siphoning of desired bacterial components or by-products.

A newer generation of geneticists, the molecular biologists, discovered that it might be possible to tinker with chromosomes without the use of mutating chemicals or radiation. To a substantial degree, they were inspired by the workings of viruses, organisms historically thought of as disease agents and as culture contaminants. Once again turning adversity into opportunity, and mimicking nature, biochemists and virologists discovered that they could follow the behavior of viruses. Many viruses seemed to be able to alter bacterial chromosomes, and indeed Lederberg was later to discover that it was possible for bacteria and viruses to swap chromosomal material. As is done by some viruses, scientists learned to unzip some particularly susceptible "extra" chromosomes present in some bacteria. These "extras" are called plasmids. Plasmids remain particularly useful even though it is now possible to patch short sequences of "foreign" genetic material into the biochemically unzipped main chromosome sequences of some bacteria as well. To a great degree, this "cutting and pasting of microbiological chromosomes" is what today's "biotechnology" and "genetic engineering" are about. And while "patch-in" chromosome sequences can be literally made by machine once the desired sequence is known, it is often only through watching microbial life cycles and analyzing what the microbes produce that clues are discovered as to what chromosome sequences are worthwhile to try and patch in.

A new perspective is that microbes, both naturally occurring and genetically engineered, are good not only for what they can be made to produce, but also for what they can dispose of. Whereas old-time "sanitary engineers" sought to find the culprits of meat or milk spoilage and destroy them, today's "bioremediation biotechnologist" is looking for bacteria that might convert garbage to useful methane or gobble up an oil spill. They actually seek to multiply those bacteria enough to clean up the environment.

## MICROBIOLOGY AND BIOTECHNOLOGY REVIEWS IN MORE GENERAL SCIENCE LITERATURE

The major multiscience journals devote review space to microbes only under certain limited circumstances. The first relates to microbes involved in very serious diseases, such as the virus that is responsible for AIDS. The second is essentially histories of the successful application of microbial technology in some highly public biotechnology venture: making "human" insulin with tailored bacteria. The third is for overviews of new mutations or techniques of chromosome manipulation that have relevance for basic science now, whether or not they will prove applicable to medicine or bioengineering later. To a substantial degree, *Science, Nature,* and the *FASEB Journal* can be selective because microbiology is correctly viewed as a reasonably mature field whose most dramatic breakthroughs are nowadays infrequent. Yet they know that microbiology cannot be held entirely in contempt-through-familiarity, given its hundreds of thousands of adherents and its sustained economic and clinical relevance.

## REVIEW SOURCES DEVOTED PRIMARILY TO MICROBIOLOGY AND BIOTECHNOLOGY

Two titles are clearly and affordably first-round review choices, suitable for even the smallest academic collections. These are *Microbiological Reviews* from the American Society for Microbiology, and the *Annual Review of Microbiology.* The former stresses exceptionally lengthy state-of-the-art reviews issued on a quarterly basis in a softbound format, the latter is the customary convenient hardbound.

The midrange collection choices are more difficult. The Euro-community is well represented by Elsevier's *FEMS Microbiological Reviews.* The U.S. has yet another softbound serial, *Critical Reviews in Microbiology* from CRC Press, and a series of solid Academic Press hardbounds, the most general of which is *Current Topics in Microbiology.* All three of these series feature a mixed review-paper/theme-issue format from time-to-time that is highly attractive. Price considerations substantially favor *Current Topics*; the citation track record gives the lead to *FEMS.* As a practical matter, if the microbiology collection would be otherwise devoid of any other European title, making the sacrifice to get this particular title now would offer substantial insights for what is still a moderate cost overall, given the importance of this discipline. The two other American titles could follow if funds allowed.

Further choices for review sources depend largely on institutional emphases in research. It is particularly important that a certain bias in "microbiology" reviews against viruses be countered. *Advances in Virus Research*, an Academic Press hardbound of roughly annual issuance is the prime source for extended reviews in the field. Fortunately, it is also very reasonable. This combination of price and quality also extends to these other Academic Press entries: *Advances in Microbial Ecology* and *Advances in Applied Microbiology*. Both feature exhaustive, state-of-the-art reviews, sometimes in thematic volumes. The latter title is probably the best established title in the field we now more commonly call "biotechnology." Biotechnology covers more than microbiology, but applied microbiology remains its core.

Three other titles in biotechnology must be considered in many locations with an industrial, pharmaceutical, or food industry orientation. *Bio/Technology* from Nature Press, while not exclusively a review journal, and indeed having a great deal of trade level information, is the first choice based on both longevity and price. The fact that *Nature* is its cousin, so to speak, has not hurt its reputation. There is a comfortable interplay between the more purely scientific and state-of-the-art reviews in *Nature* and the more practical installment and tutorial reviews in *Bio/Technology*. *Bio/Technology* is however, being strongly challenged by the highly readable and attractive *Trends in Biotechnology* from Elsevier. As with other members of this *Trends* genre, it features some of the most current minireviews, often written in tutorial style, so that nonspecialists and even some undergraduates can get a feel for events. News from the profession, conference summaries, and technical tips round out this appealing package. Its only drawback is its steep price relative to its slim monthly content, and to the rather more modest fee for *Bio/Technology*. It must remain a second choice. *Current Opinion in Biotechnology* from the U.S. publisher Current Biology is a relative newcomer to the field. It promises reviews that are not quite as exhaustive as those in *Advances in Applied Microbiology*, but are probably lengthier and more formal than those in *Bio/Technology* or in *Trends*. Some issues are thematic as well, an attractive feature. It is too soon to place a higher ranking than third or fourth on the selection list, but the author expects a rapid climb in fairly short order.

## MORE OCCASIONAL SOURCES OF MICROBIOLOGY AND BIOTECHNOLOGY REVIEWS

Since the "megareviews" have been so well handled by sources such as *Microbiological Reviews* and Academic's *Advances* series, and the midrange claimed by the *Annual Reviews*, the minireview seems fair game for many journals devoted primarily to original research. No less than fifteen significant journals feature them. They are best sorted out by generality vs. specialty.

The most general minireviews are found in the *Journal of Bacteriology* from the American Society for Microbiology, and in the *Journal of General Microbiology* from the British-based Society for General Microbiology. These titles are virtually automatic inclusions in virtually any microbiology collection, representing the best of the U.S. and the U.K., respectively. Some intensely biochemical or bacterial genetics collections might favor the aptly named "microreviews" in a new Blackwell title, *Molecular Microbiology*, as an alternative or in addition to those in the *Journal of General Microbiology*.

The choice for Continental European coverage is financially more difficult, if still straightforward. To some degree, *FEMS Microbiology Reviews* can be regarded as sufficent for smaller collections. Larger collections may want to consider *Antonie van Leeuwenhoek* from Kluwer. Not only does it feature frequent minireviews, but many life-and-times pieces. It is arguably still the journal of historical record for many European microbiologists.

The first community of specialists to be considered is the virologists. At least five sources frequently carry reviews. Two are first choices: the *Journal of Virology* from the American Society for Microbiology, and the *Journal of General Virology* from the Society for General Microbiology.

Third place is difficult, because the presence of reviews alone might not be decisive. One American title with a substantial European authorship that might qualify as a good source for intermittent reviews would be *Virology* from Academic. While it is not an inexpensive journal by any means it has a currency exchange factor advantage over Springer's *Archives of Virology*, Karger's *Intervirology*, and a number of Elsevier titles, most notably *Virus Research*. *Virology* should get the nod in most collections. For those who can afford it, one can make a selection distinction between the minireviews in *Archives of Virology* and the longer reviews in *Intervirology*. In favor of the Springer title, it should be noted that *Archives* also features a fair amount of symposia and theme papers.

The biotechnology segment deserves attention next in most collections. Three choices of intermittent review providers are once again easily made: the American Society for Microbiology's *Applied and Environmental Microbiology*, the *Journal of Applied Bacteriology* from Blackwell, and *Biotechnology and Bioengineering* from Wiley. The first favors minireviews, the second full-length state-of-the-art material, the third life-and-times material. There are two bonuses with the British title. It features a helpful "Bibliography of Reviews" section, and it covers not only biotechnology, but a fair amount of traditional "hygiene" microbiology as well.

The next level of decision making is more difficult. There are still a number of worthwhile review sources, and yet all of these remainders feature some monetary problems. *Enzyme and Microbial Technology* from Butterworth seems to feature more reviews, both minireviews and state-of-the-art, than any of its competition. Next in frequency of minireviews are those in *Letters in Applied Microbiology* from Blackwell, and in *Applied Microbiology and Biotechnology* from Springer. A final choice, particularly for wealthier libraries who wish to collect comprehensively, is *Biotechnology Letters* from Sci-Tech Letters. It is yet another minireview source.

It should be noted that *Yeast* from Wiley is the undoubted leader in tutorial reviews for this biotechnically capable microorganism.

## SYMPOSIA AND THEME ISSUES IN MICROBIOLOGY

While North American serials, including the hitherto unmentioned *Canadian Journal of Microbiology*, feature symposia and theme issues from time to time, the *Journal of Applied Bacteriology* from Blackwell, *Antonie van Leeuwenhoek* from Kluwer, and a trio of Elsevier titles feature them routinely. While the Blackwell and Kluwer titles have a fair chance of already being in many collections for reasons mentioned above, it might be wise to explore and sort out the Elsevier entries. In addition to serving as symposia sources, several may be useful for filling subject niches in your collection, if there is money. *FEMS Microbial Ecology* is the dominant Eurojournal in this field, and is a good complement to fans of *Applied and Environmental Microbiology. Research in Virology* and *Research in Microbiology* tend to feature a good deal of French "Times and Trends Symposia." That is not too surprising given that both of these journals had roots as official publications of France's historically important Pasteur Institute. French work in AIDS under Luc de Montagnier has achieved a tremendous revival of international prestige, and it is arguable that these French-based (but largely English-language) sources are worth their considerable cost.

## *METHODS LITERATURE IN MICROBIOLOGY*

Microbiology and biotechnology are blessed with methods papers in most of their general purpose journals. The identification and growing of microbial cultures, while seemingly easy in one's refrigerator, is a lot more complicated in the lab, so that more practical papers are still welcome in most journals of general microbiology. Moreover, biotechnology remains young enough that there is less agreement on standardization than might be expected of a mature field. Trade secrecy and patent protection also increasingly inhibit the sharing of detailed procedural data, so that when a research group is willing to share at least some biotechnology methods information, it becomes a matter of greater expectation and interest than in other, less commercial scientific fields.

The leaders in publishing basic microbiology methods are now the *Journal of Microbiological Methods* and the *Journal of Virological Methods*, both from Elsevier. Less obviously, but rather essentially, most collections will need the *International Journal of Systematic Bacteriology* from the American Society for Microbiology. While its longer papers are on extended schemes for sorting out families of bacteria, there are shorter technical notes concerning individual bacterial namings and corrections. Of slightly less academic standing, but having perhaps even greater biotechnical value, is *Systematic and Applied Microbiology* from VCH, a publisher better known for German chemistry.

While *Mycotaxon* from Mycotaxon Press includes many papers about large scale mushrooms, it also deals with identifying and classifiying fungal growths that are now of biotechnical importance when cultured. The leading journal for advanced work with fungi, with an increasing stress on their genetic understanding and manipulation, is, however, Academic's *Experimental Mycology*.

*Plasmid* from Wiley is essential to biotechnologists, because of the great utility of these structures in gene insertion in bacteria. Likewise, Wiley's *Yeast* remains important not only for its traditional articles on yeast breeding, physiology, and ecology, but also because it now routinely publishes "Yeast Sequencing and Mapping Reports." With these reports, both culture masters seeking to maintain uniformity, and genetic engineers looking for chromosomal segments to manipulate get a better feel for this most versatile organism.

While Wiley's *Biotechnology and Bioengineering* probably presents more methods information indirectly within its general sequence of articles than any of its competitors, a Japanese-based title, Elsevier's *Journal of Fermentation and Bioengineering,* is among the leaders in providing a regular methods section in many issues. This should not be too surprising given that the Japanese are among the world's leaders in fermented food and beverages. These traditional areas of biotechnology also support their own more practical journals, some of which should be in applied microbiology collections. Among the better known titles are the *American Journal of Enology and Viticulture* from the American Society for Enology and Viticulture, the *Journal of the American Society of Brewery Chemists*, and the *Journal of the Institute of Brewing*, a London publication. The influence of brewing on microbial genetics and biotechnology is especially evident in *Carlsberg Research Communications*, a rather prominent journal spanning many areas of cellular and molecular biology, funded by the Danish brewery whose name it bears.

# Modern General, Nuclear, and Particle Physics

While physics encompasses a vast domain of objects and force fields of all sizes, the microdomain of the nucleus, electrons, and their particles has been paramount in academic life for much of the twentieth century. Most university courses entitled "Modern Physics" are, in fact, surveys of the current state of particle physics and of the fields and forces that hold the atom together. There are basically two interacting forms of scholars in the field: theoreticians and experimentalists. Because they have a need to track one another's literature, while keeping up with their own, reviews are particularly important.

Theoretical nuclear and particle physics existed long before it was possible to actually track and characterize most individual particles experimentally. Theoretical physics is historically a profession for widely scattered "loners" or small working groups who tend to think, speak, and publish in highly mathematical terms. Predicting particle properties and behavior (important for recognizing when new particles have made an appearance in an experimental detector) or uncovering consistent patterns among scattered reports of particles from recent experiments keeps theorists busy in their offices and our libraries. It is safe to say that there are many more theoretical papers on particles than particles. The greatest multiplier of papers is not the number of suspected but still unknown particles, or their often extremely short lifespans and rapid transformations, but rather the number of theoreticians alive and revising their models at any given moment.

[Haworth co-indexing entry note]: "Modern General, Nuclear, and Particle Physics." Stankus, Tony. Co-published simultaneously in *The Serials Librarian* (The Haworth Press, Inc.) Vol. 27, No. 2/3, 1995, pp. 143-152; and: *Special Format Serials and Issues: Annual Review of . . . , Advances in . . . , Symposia on . . . , Methods in . . .* (ed: Tony Stankus) The Haworth Press, Inc., 1995, pp. 143-152. Single or multiple copies of this article are available from The Haworth Document Delivery Service [1-800-342-9678, 9:00 a.m. - 5:00 p.m. (EST)].

*143*

Experimentalists, by contrast, write fewer papers, and do so in giant teams of over two hundred coauthors. They gather at perhaps a dozen sites around the world. Such enormous teams exist for two reasons. It often takes that many scientists to run the gigantic accelerators that smash atoms into particles. It may take even more to read all those papers from the theoretical physicists after the last experiment and before the next.

## REVIEWS IN MODERN GENERAL, NUCLEAR, AND PARTICLE PHYSICS IN MULTISCIENCE JOURNALS

The discovery of a new particle or the proposal of a particularly promising model for a family of particles is treated as an event of Nobel Prize-winning proportions. While the use of the broadcast media to make such pronouncements is still frowned upon as grandstanding, a useful analogy may be the two-step still seen on TV: "This late-breaking news . . . (followed by a sketchy announcement) . . . with details at eleven." The initial announcements tend to be published as brief, rapid communications in one of the holy trinity of *Physical Review Letters*, *Physics Letters*, or *Europhysics Letters*. The list of authors in the letters journals literally exceeds the word count of the text in many cases. The details appear later as state-of-the-art reviews in *Science* and *Nature*, with only the team leaders generally serving as authors. One also finds additional tutorial reviews in the "News and Views" sections, composed by their permanent editorial staffs, for neophytes.

## REVIEWS IN MODERN GENERAL, NUCLEAR, AND PARTICLE PHYSICS IN GENERAL PURPOSE PHYSICS JOURNALS

The major scientific powers in physics have developed such a strong network of stand-alone journals for reviews that few general purpose physics journals carry them on a regular basis. The central question in collection management for this field is which of the many review vehicles one ought to take, and whether or not to stress general physics reviews or particle physics reviews. It is nonetheless wise to check on the few exceptions to the stand-alone review journals.

The most prominent exception by far, is Academic's *Annals of Physics.* While the "New York" *Annals*–so called, to distinguish it from the French *Annales* and the German *Annalen*–was designed as a vehicle for lengthy original research papers, it has become de facto one of the principal English language outlets for papers that have very substantial literature reviews and intellectual histories of the concepts being explored. The bulk of the papers in any issue have a strong review character.

There are other journals from major powers that make an occasional exception. The brief communications journal *Progress of Theoretical Physics* (Tokyo) publishes supplements that contain review papers. One reason why this is important is historical: Japanese workers were distinguished in the past for work in mesons, an important category of particles, still under much debate. The other reason is current: Japanese accelerators, while not the largest in the world, are among the newest and best supported financially. Despite its *Theoretical* title, recent experimental data is often incorporated.

The *Journal of Physics* series from the (British) Institute of Physics will have reviews from time-to-time, even if they are not prominently headlined as reviews. This same is true for the *Canadian Journal of Physics.* Neither of these countries, however, is particularly noted for large resident accelerators so much as for a continuing tradition of good theoretical workers.

Ironically, the frequency of reviews in the remaining national physics journals tends to increase with a decrease in their national overall scientific standing. This means that the physics journals of Third World countries and even some other rising Asian powers include reviews much more often than do those of major western scientific powers. It might be noted, for example, that the *International Journal of Modern Physics, Section A*, a nascent star from World Scientific Publishers in Singapore, features an extensive review in most issues, as does *Pramana*, a well-established physics journal from India. Most of these reviews are state-of-the-art by intention, but their authors frequently show less contact with the latest trends, reducing their currency and worldwide influence.

Yet another exception should be noted. Certain journals from major western scientific powers that mix research and teaching functions welcome tutorial reviews. For example, the *American Journal of Physics*, and its Continental counterpart, the *European Journal of Physics*, are vehicles for reviews aimed at the more sophisticated college instructor in the field. They publish a fair number of life-and-times reviews in which the collective biography of an historically important development is often tied in with the explication of a pedagogically difficult concept. This is also true in a number of semi-popular general physics journals, although most of their pieces are minireviews. *Physics Today* from the American Physical Society is one example. That title also features extended obituaries which function very much like life-and-times minireviews. Continental European journals follow suit with even more and longer death notices of major national physics figures, commonly including commentary on their major papers. *Contemporary Physics* from Taylor and Francis is less biographical in its reviews. It is effectively a journal for highly readable tutorials, a kind of *Scientific American* exclusively devoted to physics as affecting daily life or industry.

Finally, a great many papers by mathematical physicists, written in either journals of general physics or in journals of applied mathematics, have a strong formal tutorial character. This is partly due to the fact that the flow of new models in particle physics tends to come from areas of mathematics, like differential geometry and topology, that have developed a terminology of their own which must be translated and explicated for working physicists. There is also a life-and-times component to some of these papers because of the strong attachment of mathematicians to eponyms–technical terms whose inventor's name is often attached. A substantial portion of theoretical physics and terminology is still tied to pioneers in the field: Einstein, Bohr, Dirac, Bose, Fermi, etc., with allusions to their more general theories quite common in the names of particles, fields or effects.

## SERIALS DEVOTED TO REVIEWS IN MODERN GENERAL, NUCLEAR, AND PARTICLE PHYSICS

The overwhelming source for extended perspectives in modern physics, however, comes from serials devoted solely to reviews.

Fortunately, they can be ranked in discrete tiers of leadership, and sorted by a "general" versus "specifically particle" spin. Interestingly, the top tier, even for heavy particle concentrators, is nominally "general," but these, in fact, publish a great many of the most important reviews in nuclear and particle physics. These include the *Reviews of Modern Physics* from the American Institute of Physics, *Reports on the Progress of Physics* from the (British) Institute of Physics, and *Physics Reports* from Elsevier. All three are soft-bound, and favor state-of-the-art reviews with some life-and-times detail.

There are some important distinctions of publishing strategies between the first two serials and the third, however. While the first, *Reviews of Modern Physics*, is a full format quarterly, and the second, *Reports on the Progress of Physics*, a more compact monthly, both generally feature a number of different papers in each issue. *Physics Reports*, by contrast, consists of individually issued and jacketed review papers: each issue consists of a single paper, each paper is an entire issue. This is done both to expedite the publication of each review as it is ready, and to allow Elsevier to sell the individual papers as a form of second-wind cost recovery. The latter consideration is not trivial financially. *Physics Reports* is the review companion to one of the most expensive rapid communications journals, *Physics Letters A and B*, and is itself the most expensive review serial mentioned in this chapter. Many libraries that would like ready access to the complete run of this review probably cannot afford it, but will purchase important single issues.

Assuming that the collection manager can afford to take all three of these, what is the best strategy for any remaining money? Does he or she opt for the next tier of nominally general modern physics reviews, or collect more obviously dedicated nuclear and particle titles? To a degree, the amount of local emphasis on nuclear and particles physics may provide an answer. If it is moderate as opposed to intense, then two additional general physics reviews are recommended. The readers will still get a good deal of nuclear and particle information while having access to other topics as well.

The second tier of more general physics reviews includes *Annales de Physique* from Editions Physique, and *Rivista del Nuovo Cimento*, from the Italian Physical Society. While lengthy state-of-the-art reviews are nominally the chief fare of these journals, there is a substantial amount of life-and-times detail in many papers. Each of these second tier titles has had an historical or cultural background that has influenced its current standing as a review today.

The French entry, the *Annales de Physique* has benefited from the remarkable transformation of one of its sister publications, and actually increased its standing in recent years. Editions Physique, publisher of *Annales*, scored a major coup when it took over management of an Italian journal of physics of some international standing, *Lettere al Nuovo Cimento*. The French merged it with their own *Journal de Physique, Lettres* to create the highly successful *Europhysics Letters*. As mentioned above, *Europhysics Letters* has become one of the three must-buy journals for announcements in high energy particle experimentation. To some degree then, *Annales de Physique* is the review closest to *Europhysics Letters*. This affiliation would be decisive save for two factors: its Italian partner still functions independently when it comes to reviews; and some *Annales* papers continue to appear in French. The latter factor is not as much a collection disqualification as might be expected. The greatest strength of French physics has been on the mathematical and theoretical side, and mathematicians are among the few remaining Americans with a science Ph.D. training that still requires some reading ability in French.

This brings us to *Rivista del Nuovo Cimento*, an almost completely English-language serial. The Italian tradition in experimental nuclear and particle physics has historically been very strong, given the tradition of Nobel Prize-winners such as Fermi and Segre, albeit many of its best scholars emigrated to the U.S. to do their best work. Some would argue that the migration of *Lettere* to French administration was a kind of added misfortune for the Italian Physical Society as well. But the loss for the Italians has been more apparent than real. The Italian Society maintains some role in *Lettere*'s functioning as *Europhysics Letters*. This transformation represents more of a successful Pan-Europeanization or Internationalization of Italian physics journals than a decline, and *Rivista* shares in this export-derived prestige. *Rivista* has been designated an official "Europhysics" journal by a consortium of Continental societies. Despite its relatively high status, *Rivista* remains a highly affordable outlet for reviews. (The lira is, thankfully for American buyers, a generally weak currency.) And at least partly because of its higher proportion of English-language papers, it attracts a greater number of American authors than its French competitor.

This brings the reader to the alternative strategy: a second tier that frankly concentrates nuclear and particle work. Fortunately, there are three clearcut selections at this tier, and an optional fourth title.

The survey of first choice is Plenum's *Advances in Nuclear Physics*. A somewhat irregular "annual," it generally features the fewest, but also the longest and most heavily cited state-of-the-art reviews. The *Annual Review of Nuclear and Particle Science* competes quite well. It has clocklike regularity, and has more papers per volume, of intermediate length and with highly respectable citation rates. Moreover, it is, by far, the best selection in cost factors. A highly complementary, and more strongly European focus and authorship is represented in Pergamon's *Progress in Particle and Nuclear Physics*, a work which typically encompasses two hard volumes a year. Together, these three serials cost about the same as the second tier of French and Italian titles mentioned above, and at least the *Annual Review* could well be afforded in about any collection scheme. Some collections may also wish to consider the more informal reviews found in Gordon and Breach's *Comments on Nuclear and Particle Physics*. While it has not made the impact of other titles in this cluster, its added cost is not particularly onerous.

## SYMPOSIA AND THEME JOURNALS IN MODERN AND PARTICLE PHYSICS

Physics is awash in scientific congresses, and a great many symposia are organized seemingly ad hoc with proceedings published on a somewhat unpredictable schedule afterward. Fortunately, many of the more established, recurring symposia treat topics pertinent to nuclei, particles, and the accompanying mathematics at least annually, and often even more frequently. The first choices are the *AIP Conference Proceedings Series*, the (British) *Institute of Physics Conference Series Proceedings*, and the *NATO Advanced Stud-*

*ies Institutes: Series B: Physics.* They draw their strength through a combination of prestige and a better organizational machinery for raising corporate support and more reliable publication. Taking the whole of these three series in order to ensure prompt arrival of individually pertinent volumes may well be worth it, given standing order discounts and uniformly high quality. Selections of symposia after these three flagships involve greater uncertainties of timely arrival, quality, and sufficient emphasis on nuclear and particle work.

In most other cases, an item-by-item approach would be better. For a variety of factors, this selective approach is also often the only one possible. It should be noted that few conferences in modern physics, other than these three, have a consistent corporate author name, or uniform main entry, making their tracking for acquisitions and cataloging problematic. Rather, they are known to their physics readers largely through the site where they are held or by the historical figure in whose honor they are convened. Shifts in publisher within a given conference series are rather common. No less than six firms have at times published short stretches of the series to be discussed shortly. These publishers include Plenum, Gordon and Breach, World Scientific, Elsevier, and Academic, and now Wolters Kluwer. Most of these "other" conference proceedings are hardbound, some with a finished, typeset format, but more and more publishers are using a camera-ready-copy format for them. Springer also handles some of these as *Lecture Notes in Physics,* a softbound series, generally using camera-ready-copy format. (The Springer series also includes a number of other worthwhile conferences not detailed here.)

Among the more prominent conferences are the so-called "Summer Schools," typically held at resort areas in Europe. These are partly post-doctoral seminars with some classroom instruction by an international assortment of star speakers, and partly regular conferences with presentations by lesser-known physicists. In most cases, it is only the work of the invited speakers that is printed in full. The leading French work is seen in the *Les Houches* series (based on summer schools at the University of Grenoble, near les Houches, an Alpine hotel) and the *Cargese* series (based on summer school at Cargese, a resort on the isle of Corsica). The Italians sponsor equally prominent summer symposia: the *Trieste* series (named after the Adriatic resort), *Enrico Fermi* series (named after the Nobel Prize-winner and held at Verona), and the *Ettore Majorana* series (named after a colleague of Fermi's who died an untimely death; held at the port of Erice in Sicily). It should be noted that in the 1980s, an exceptional number of independent conferences in Europe, North America, and the Pacific Rim have been handled by World Scientific, the Singapore publisher, and that a consultation of their catalog is apt to prove rewarding as a means of tracking these conferences.

Theme issue journals in modern physics are fairly rare. Almost alone among major general purpose physics journals, *Physica Scripta* from the Swedish Academy of Sciences on behalf of a Scandinavian consortium, features them regularly, and a number are pertinent to modern nuclear and particle physics. The Springer series *Lecture Notes in Physics,* mentioned as a source for conference proceedings, has a number of issues that have substantial likelihood of being effectively theme-issues. The "conference" papers they contain have been substantially reworked, and the entire conference has been broken up into separately issued notebooks of like-minded talks so that the final products frequently resemble theme issues.

## METHODS SERIALS IN MODERN NUCLEAR AND PARTICLE PHYSICS

A number of *Handbuch*-like treatises in physics have sections that are devoted to methods. The most important of these is Academic's *Methods of Experimental Physics*, a hardbound revised periodically (Volume 2B is the most pertinent). Academic is also responsible for *Atomic Data and Nuclear Data Tables*, an ongoing series of experimental values obtained under carefully detailed conditions. Most experimental workers, however, will place heavier emphasis on three more frequently issued serials.

The leaders, in decreasing order of prominence, are: *Nuclear Instruments and Methods in Physics Research* from Elsevier, *IEEE Transactions on Nuclear Science*, and *Particle Accelerators* from Gordon and Breach. It should be acknowledged immediately that the first title is frightfully expensive, but it must be remembered that its core readership is people at facilities with budgets in the tens of millions of dollars, at the minimum. The slant of the journal is more towards the physicists than to the army of engineers that assist them at accelerator facilties. The reasonable price for the second publication is owing to its being much smaller, but nonetheless one of a large family of titles fielded by the IEEE, the leading organization for the well-supported field of electronics and electrical engineering. The slant of this journal is clearly towards the technical support professionals who help the experiments go. The Gordon and Breach publication, *Particle Accelerators*, is closer in both price and orientation to the Elsevier publication. Its status might be higher save for some problems of frequency, and the fact that its competitors are perceived already to be quite capable and comprehensive.

# The Neurosciences

The 1990s are the "Decade of the Brain," and both fundamental and clinical neurosciences can be expected to blossom. There are over 20,000 members of the Society for Neuroscience, and this figure does not include many clinical neurologists or neurosurgeons who have their own organizations. Federal funding for studies of the brain, its diseases, and the biological basis of behavior, will be at least half a billion dollars annually until the year 2000.

The neurosciences are one of the most subdivided fields represented in this book. Even the classification of clinical vs. fundamental neurosciences represents only the first sorting.

Hospital-based specialties might be further broken down into noninvasive neurology, neurosurgery, medical imaging of the brain and nervous system, psychiatry with psychopharmacology, as well as allied health sciences (some diagnostic, and some rehabilitative).

University campus specialties within neuroscience typically involve several departments. There is the chemistry of natural neurotransmitters as well as the synthesis and laboratory manipulation of drugs affecting the nervous system. Biology departments generally have charge of in vitro molecular and cellular neuroscience, as well as comparative neuroanatomy and neurophysiology. Psychology contributes cognitive neuropsychology, perceptual psychophysics and laboratory-based studies of learning and behavior. Departments of psychology and biology either fight over, or share, "psychobiology," the study of the biological basis of complex behavior. In some institutions, animal behavior experts from the zoology department called "ethologists" tend to dominate psychobiology. In oth-

[Haworth co-indexing entry note]: "The Neurosciences." Stankus, Tony. Co-published simultaneously in *The Serials Librarian* (The Haworth Press, Inc.) Vol. 27, No. 2/3, 1995, pp. 153-162; and: *Special Format Serials and Issues: Annual Review of . . . , Advances in . . . , Symposia on . . . , Methods in . . .* (ed: Tony Stankus) The Haworth Press, Inc., 1995, pp. 153-162. Single or multiple copies of this article are available from The Haworth Document Delivery Service [1-800-342-9678, 9:00 a.m. - 5:00 p.m. (EST)].

*153*

ers, specialists within psychology called "physiological psychologists" hold sway. Computer science departments have entered the fray with neural network modelling. Even philosophy and language studies contribute academic cognitive science and neurolinguistics.

The boundaries of clinical vs. fundamental neurosciences can be crossed from time to time, and certain coalitions are common. Noninvasive neurologists tend to rely on cognitive neuropsychologists to evaluate deficits in thinking, speaking, writing, and task completion in patients who have had some neurological misadventure. Psychiatrists need a good deal of information from the neurochemical community in order to understand the modes of action of given psychotropic drugs. Neurosurgeons and rehabilitative physicians (physiatrists) even now seek to gauge just how much motor loss a given invasive procedure is likely to engender, based partly on studies of animals (comparative neuroanatomy and neurophysiology) in the hopes of salvaging some function, or allowing for some rerouting of signal processing. Moreover, some tremor-engendering diseases like Parkinsonism seem to respond to surgical implants of tissue cultures of fetal material (the domain of in vitro molecular and cellular neuroscience). Nonetheless, some distinctions in professional reading habits and information seeking practices will remain for some time to come, partly because the medical and basic science communities still have somewhat segregated educational pathways and differing publishing houses.

## REVIEWS OF THE NEUROSCIENCES
## IN MULTISCIENCE JOURNALS

Neurosciences are scientifically "hot." Reviews in multiscience journals like *Science* and *Nature* dealing with the more fundamental neurosciences are not unusual. Molecular and cellular neurosciences fare the best, clinical neurosurgery and rehabilitative subjects do more poorly. Perceptual psychology and animal behavior actually do better than clinical topics, largely because the editors of *Science* and *Nature* understand that academic psychologists and zoologists are more loyal readers of these journals than are medical doctors. Minireviews in *Cell* remain important for the more molecular neurosciences although, since its sister journal *Neuron* has come upon the scene, they are somewhat less common. The *FASEB Journal* has a fair amount of review material in regulatory and integrative neurophysiology (the brain as a coordinator of bodily function and movement). Despite the appearance of many reviews in these multiscience outlets, the bulk of neuroscience reviewing goes into journals more or less exclusively devoted to them.

## SOURCES DEVOTED TO NEUROSCIENCE

Basic neuroscience leads medical neurology by far in the provision of separate vehicles for reviews. Even two nominally general neuroscience reviews are in fact, heavily fundamental, although still quite worth taking in many larger clinical collections. The *Annual Review of Neuroscience* from the not-for-profit Annual Reviews, Inc., is a bargain featuring very high quality papers, usually of an intermediate length and state-of-the-art survey type. It is almost always the most cited serial within this field and appeals to a wide range of established professionals and academics. It belongs in every library within any constituency of neuroscience.

*Trends in Neuroscience* from Elsevier has been chasing the *Annual Reviews* for several years, and is closing the gap somewhat. It offers highly readable minireviews on a monthly basis, many of them approachable by nonspecialists, although generally written by leaders in the field. Illustrated, containing news and announcements as well as reviews, it is clearly the fastest way to get up to speed in many new developments. Its price is a drawback, costing a few hundred where the *Annual Reviews* still comes in at less than one hundred. Nonetheless, it is clearly the very next choice in most collections.

Choices become less universal as we go down the list. *Brain Research Reviews*, also from Elsevier, is a special section remaining from the breakdown of the massive leader of the 1970s, *Brain Research*. This journal has strengths with neuroanatomists, neurophysiologists, and psychopharmacologists. (This coalition of specialists is explained by the use of special markers to establish the sites of action, within the brain, of given drugs.) While it still remains relatively expensive, in the few hundreds of dollars range, this is a major improvement in affordability over the old consolidated journal.

*Progress in Neurobiology* has strong ties to the neurophysiology community with some appeal to the psychobiology contingent. The psychobiology community is more exclusively served in *Neuroscience and Biobehavioral Reviews*. These latter two journals share a publisher, Pergamon, and a propensity for very long, authoritative state-of-the-art essays. While they might be overlooked in collection policies for small libraries, owing to a cost in the several hundreds, they ought to be taken in any institution with a graduate program in physiology or psychology.

Somewhat similar in scope to these two publications, but hardbound and substantially less expensive, are two Academic Press irregulars. These are *Progress in Psychobiology and Physiological Psychology*, the most closely matching title, and *Advances in the Study of Behavior*, a title that has both psychobiology and ethology loyalties. These are certainly acceptable substitutes for smaller collections. A bonus is that some of their issues are thematic review issues, combining two functions, extended survey work and multiple viewpoints, in one.

Clinical neurosciences have finally gotten their due with the arrival of *Current Opinion in Neurology and Neurosurgery* from Current Science. Current Science has long been moving in on Elsevier's *Trends* series with a slightly higher level paper, longer bibliographies, and a fair number of theme issues. It should be interesting to see if its reviews are more cited than those found in the leading clinical journals, which have concentrated most of the clinical survey functions within their covers. Another clinical survey journal is more specialized. *Cerebrovascular and Brain Metabolism Reviews* comes to us from Raven, arguably the most important publisher of specialized clinical journals in neurology. Its scope is somewhat larger than stroke (the principal cerebrovascular mishap) and its future is also bright in that MRI (magnetic resonance imaging) and PET (positron emission tomography) are making great strides in allowing the visualization of blood flow and brain nutrient and chemical processing.

Psychopharmacology is in a privileged position in brain research. Research into practical medicines relating to the human nervous system and mental disorders is well-supported by the clinical community for reasons of both altruism and exceptional economic reward. (Tranquilizers and antidepressants are perenially atop the lists of the world's most prescribed drugs.) Pharmacological approaches are also extremely popular for studying animal brain metabolism and behavior in nonclinical research settings. Basic science centers frequently receive financial support and gifts of experimental drugs from pharmaceutical firms in return for access to research results that may be useful in documenting the safety or efficacy of some new medicine. Pharmacological papers are welcome in many basic reviews of the brain sciences and in reviews for psychiatrists. The *Annual of Pharmacology and Toxicology* almost always has about 20% "psycho-or-neuro" papers. The leading review source specifically devoted to the juncture between basic and clinical work in this field appears to be *Advances in Biochemical Psychopharmacology*, an annual from Raven, earlier noted as one of the leading neurology publishers in the country.

## REGULAR NEUROSCIENCE JOURNALS AS REVIEW SOURCES

If basic sciences led among journals devoted to reviews, clinical neurosciences dominate in having reviews within the mainstream of their general purpose journals. Each of the "Big Three" of clinical neurology features them regularly. *Neurology*, from Edgell Communications, has both frequent formal state-of-the-art "Reviews," as well as a plethora of more occasional "Issues" or "Views" (current controversies) and "Special" and "Invited" articles. Each of these less regular types tends to be shorter, some are minireviews, and it is common for each to have some editorial comment. *Neurology* also has "Historical Neurology," brief notes of a life-and-times character. *Archives of Neurology* from the AMA has an equally impressive array. Its more formal articles are presented as "Neurological Reviews," but "Special Articles," "Minireviews," "Editorials," and "Controversies" are quite common. Like *Neurology*, the *Archives* has a "History of Medicine" feature. The *Annals of Neurology* from Little-Brown, has fewer reviews than its peers, but still a great many relative to journals serving more basic neurosciences. Its more comprehensive reviews are produced under the heading "Neurological Progress." Shorter are "Brief Reviews," "Editorials," and historical "Vignettes."

Other American outlets for clinicians are similar. The *Journal of Neuropathology and Experimental Neurology* from Raven for the American Association of Neuropathology, features regular state of the art "Reviews," as well as life-and-times pieces, and extremely large population case reviews and meta-analyses. *Neurosurgery* from William and Wilkins features some state-of-the-art reviews, and fairly frequent "Historical Articles." *Movement Disorders* from Raven has both a "Viewpoint" editorial minireview series, and regular reviews. *Metabolic Brain Diseases* from Academic follows much the same pattern: brief editorial reviews and lengthier surveys.

Psychiatry, psychopharmacology, and behavioral neuropharmacology, have a vast and increasingly intertwined literature, and only a few of their most important general purpose journals having reviews will be mentioned here. These were selected at least partly for having some reviews that substantially involve drugs and neurobiological approaches, as opposed to a stress on purely psychosocial issues or talk therapies alone. The most important American leaders include the *Archives of General Psychiatry* from the American Medical Association. It features both "News and Views" pieces, which tend towards minireviews, and "Perspectives," which can have either a contemporary "minireview" or a life-and-times approach. The *American Journal of Psychiatry* from the American Psychiatric Association tends to feature "Special Articles" and longer "Reviews" that frequently stress meta-analyses of drug trials. The case is similar with the *Journal of Nervous and Mental Diseases* from Williams and Wilkins, although their reviews are somewhat less numerous.

*Clinical Neuropharmacology* from Raven has become the number one specialty journal for drug-prescribing neurologists. The importance of its state-of-the art reviews is second only to those in the "Big Three" general purpose neurology journals mentioned earlier.

The foreign clinical press also features reviews among general purpose articles, although not nearly so many as their American counterparts. The most numerous appear in the British Medical Association's *Journal of Neurology, Neurosurgery, and Psychiatry.*

Most are "Editorial Reviews." From Cambridge University Press, we have *Developmental Medicine and Child Neurology*. It has both brief "Annotations," and longer overviews.

On the Continent, Elsevier's *Journal of the Neurological Sciences* features highlighted "Editorial Reviews" (which are characteristically briefer) as well as more conventional state-of-the-art reviews of some length, appearing alongside papers of regular research. Springer's *Journal of Neurology* has a regular "News and Views" section, essentially a running installment series of minireviews. *Child's Nervous System* is another Springer entry. It has somewhat more frequent regular reviews, as well as biographical pieces, and an annual "Presidential Address," which can have either a life-and-times or installment review character. Still another Springer title, *Acta Neuropathologica* confines its reviewing largely to straightforward state-of-the-art work. Karger, a major Swiss biomedical firm, offers *Cerebrovascular Diseases*, with intermittent state-of-the-art reviews.

The number of journals in the more basic neurosciences with reviews is substantially smaller. Number one in terms of molecular and cellular importance are the "minireviews" in *Neuron* from Cell Press. Closely following are the lengthier state-of-the-art reviews in the *Journal of Neuroscience* from the Society for Neuroscience, and the "Commentary" critical minireviews section of *Neuroscience* from Pergamon. Academic Press has combined these features by having both full-length surveys and "Commentary" minireviews in its *Molecular and Cellular Neurosciences*.

The chemistry community relies primarily on "Short Reviews" in Raven's *Journal of Neurochemistry*, and on longer "Invited Reviews" in Pergamon's *Neurochemistry International*.

Physiologists still see some neurophysiology reviews in the major reviews journal of general physiology. Their frequency and importance for neurophysiologists falls roughly in this order: *Annual Review of Physiology*, *Physiological Reviews*, *News in the Physiological Sciences*. But more and more neurophysiology, particularly electroneurophysiology reviews are appearing in vehicles like Elsevier's *Neuroscience Research* and in Springer's *Journal of Neural Transmission*. The latter contains substantial reviews of disordered neural impulses and surveys attempts at their clinical management, often with drug therapy.

The neuropsychology contingent has two main outlets that contain intermittent reviews: *Brain and Cognition* from Academic and the *Journal of Cognitive Neuroscience* from MIT. Both feature state-of-the-art reviews, with a more clinical "head injury" orientation in the former vehicle and a more theoretical, academic bent in the latter.

## SYMPOSIA AND THEME ISSUES
## IN THE NEUROSCIENCES

In America and in Europe, both clinicians and basic scientists meet often for conferences in the neurosciences, sometimes jointly but more often separately. American journals, whether basic or clinical, tend to emphasize only the major speeches. These plenary talks are turned, often with strong editorial guidance, into quasi-review papers of the installment-type. These are published on an intermittent basis, with perhaps a discreet footnote indicating their oral origin. European journals, whether basic or clinical, tend to carry many more talks but without much editing. By contrast with the Americans, they tend to cluster the talks together in a conference issue and thereby highlight their connection to the event. European journals with symposia talks clearly tend to outnumber those of a U.S. symposium or thematic origin.

The leading thematic/symposia sources in American neurosciences are the *Neurological Clinics* from Saunders, and *Behavioral and Brain Sciences* from Cambridge University Press. The former is a highly conservative collection of review-type essays generally centered around an announced theme. It strongly appeals to practicing neurologists and neurosurgeons, and is recommended for even small hospital collections with attending neurologists. The latter publication, by contrast, is a freewheeling invention comprised of a few lengthy, often provocative papers, with each followed by up to two dozen brief, and generally sharp, signed commentaries and critiques. This procedure sometimes yields "heckling in print," but in any case represents the staging of a lively if vicarious debate as is encountered in any literature. The principal audience for *Behavioral and Brain Sciences* is academic and its slant is primarily neuro-psychological, although papers from ethologists and experimental psychologists can be found often enough to make its inclusion in most university collections readily justified.

Two others among the few American journals which pay attention to conferences are the clinical *Neurology*, and the basic science *Cellular and Molecular Neurobiology* from Plenum. The first, which contains selective reporting, is an automatic choice for a variety of reasons; the second has not yet achieved such standing, although it often features more and lengthier conference pieces. The *Journal of Neuroscience*, another automatic choice for reasons other than its conference coverage, also publishes the *Society for Neuroscience Abstracts*, an annual now in two volumes of about 10,000 summaries for a single convention.

The European array is not only larger but more varied. Live symposia talks and conference overviews are not only frequent in largely clinical vehicles such as Springer's *Journal of Neurology and Psychopharmacology* but also in a broad array of Elsevier and Karger titles. The Dutch firm features special issues in *Electroencephalography and Clinical Neurophysiology, Neuropsychopharmacology*, and *Schizophrenia Research*. Elsevier's Pergamon partner further fields *Neurochemistry International, Neurotoxicology and Teratology*, and *Psychoneuroendocrinology*, all of which have theme issues, symposia, and *festchrifts*. Karger is notable in this regard for *Developmental Neuroscience, Cerebrovascular Diseases*, and *Neuroepidemiology*. Thieme, a German publisher, is notable for "theme" issues, in its *Pharmacopsychiatry. Neurotoxicology*, from Intox, publishes the proceedings of the International Neurotoxicity Association.

Commonwealth countries are intermediate between American and European attitudes on symposia and themes. The *Canadian Journal of Neurological Sciences* from the National Research Council irregularly includes symposia supplements, as does the *Journal of Neurology, Neurosurgery, and Psychiatry* from the British Medical Association. It should be frankly stated that none of these Continental or Commonwealth journals should rise and fall solely on their conference or theme issues, and no general "must buy" recommendation can be given. The best strategy in a larger collection would

be to initially prefer those conference-rich journals that most closely match the most active segments of your neuroscience community, before taking any titles that are somewhat more marginal to local
interests.


## SOURCES OF METHODS IN THE NEUROSCIENCES

To a substantial degree, most clinical journals, especially in surgery and in medical imaging, are essentially journals of method.
Virtually no titles in this category are without papers involving
great procedural detail. Nervous system electrophysiology, because
of its long history and enormous utility in human diagnosis, is well
supported and documented even when it is applied to laboratory
animals.

The characteristic difficulty of neuroscience literature has typically been finding sources of methods in the more basic neurosciences. This stems from the fact that until recently, molecular and
cellular neuroscience technical notes were treated as one subset
among many in journals of biochemistry and tissue culture. This
has changed dramatically in the last several years, and three titles
have appeared which concentrate the best work in the field.

The seniormost and most voluminous has been Elsevier's *Journal of Neuroscience Methods*. It publishes approximately three
times as many papers as its newer competitors, but costs about five
times as much. Featuring full-length papers, it remains the journal
of choice, and is recommended for all large collections. The two
newer entries are at opposite ends of the size-of-entry spectrum: the
regular softbound *NeuroProtocols* is typically composed of shorter
notes while *Methods in Neurosciences* is an irregular hardbound
series of lengthier pieces usually focused on a single theme. These
approaches are somewhat complementary and this arrangement is
probably by design of their common publisher, Academic. Every
collection of academic neuroscience should have this pair, once it
has secured the Elsevier entry. The early promise of the Academic
entry is such that unless Elsevier prevents defections from among
their American contributors and does some price-cutting as well,
this recommendation may be reversed.

# Oceans, Atmosphere, Weather, and Climate

Geophysical scientists have come to see the earth's water and air as a continuum. For them, weather is an ongoing swirling interaction between atmospheric and ocean currents. The largest source of the stirring energy is the earth's own rotation. But solar radiation, heat reflected from the earth's surface, and even the tidal pull of the moon add significantly. Consequences of ocean-air swirling can be seen even far inland, on local (microscale), regional (mesoscale), and even continental (synoptic) scales.

Some massive ocean-air episodes might occur once a decade. Currents such as El Nino trap solar radiation more intensely in a given year, changing ocean-air patterns in the South Pacific. Moist cyclonic circulation goes where it shouldn't be, and may generate uncharacteristic floods as far away as Texas for months at a time, while impoverishing cold-water fishing off the coast of Chile.

Phenomena that we take as seasonal often involve a complex cycle of air-land-and-water interactions. In summertime, clashes of energized hot and cold fronts in the Far West generate lightning storms. These ignite massive forest fires in dried timberlands. The resulting firestorms propel smoke high into the atmosphere with plumes extending hundreds of miles downwind. Water droplets high in the atmosphere achieve a certain critical mass by collectively clinging to the suspended soot, leading to severe downpours in the midwest. Factories in the midwest that burn high sulfur coal begin the long range cycle again. Sulfrous particles and vapors from

[Haworth co-indexing entry note]: "Oceans, Atmosphere, Weather, and Climate." Stankus, Tony. Co-published simultaneously in *The Serials Librarian* (The Haworth Press, Inc.) Vol. 27, No. 2/3, 1995, pp. 163-170; and: *Special Format Serials and Issues: Annual Review of . . . , Advances in . . . , Symposia on . . . , Methods in . . .* (ed: Tony Stankus) The Haworth Press, Inc., 1995, pp. 163-170. Single or multiple copies of this article are available from The Haworth Document Delivery Service [1-800-342-9678, 9:00 a.m. - 5:00 p.m. (EST)].

their smokestacks generate droplets of acid rain over New England and Eastern Canada.

Instances of ocean-air interaction can also occur daily: inversions of the atmosphere over a major coastal city like Los Angeles result in a smog cap. While there are a number of ways that the cap can be popped, the most refreshing involve cold, ocean-current-driven winds. (The desert-roasted Santa Ana winds will also do the job, albeit much less comfortably.)

Even relatively remote, long term, upper atmospheric phenomena have come into the news. People fear the penetration of more solar UV rays through holes in the ozone layer. Will humans get more skin cancer, and other animals or plants be adversely affected? Others wonder about the warming effect of greenhouse gases. Will the polar ice caps melt at an abnormally high rate, resulting in a raising of sea levels and increased coastal flooding? Are these exaggerated fears? Have these things happened before? What can the records of the earth's past tell us about the planet's response to a changing environment? We now know that the massive eruption of Mount Pinatubo in the Phillipines in 1991, which injected enormous amounts of gases and ash high into the upper atmosphere, probably is responsible for a cooling effect of a degree or two for the following year. But can we count on volcanoes as a relief valve for an overheated planet? What has been the actual temperature of the earth during the last 100 years or 10,000 years? Such conundrums consitute the interpretive lot of the climatological segment of this continuum of oceanic and atmospheric scientists.

Not all of the interest in ocean and atmospheric reactions is driven by practical concerns over weather or the environment. Much is essentially academic and no application is expected, while some fluid behavior analysis is applied in unexpected ways by scientists who seem quite distant in specialty. Mathematical physicists are a prime example. They have long grappled with describing the behavior of gases or liquids into workable equations. Fluid engineers are yet another example. They typically come from chemical engineering industries that involve processing large quantities of liquids and gases, and join their purely academic colleagues in this interest in fluid behaviors. They need to know when things are likely to get out of hand in a big reaction vessel or while mixing pipeline flows. Both theoretical models, and workplace experiences, have shown that gases and liquids share surprisingly complex behaviors like streaming, turbulence, vortexes, percolation, and convection. Perhaps it is not surprising that there is much unification of gas and liquid models. This conceptual unification has resulted in the specialty of fluid mechanics or fluid dynamics. The fluid mechanics-dynamics contingent looks upon the earth's air-ocean continuum as a particularly challenging, but sometimes obliging drama that plays out scenarios in which scientists can be both participants and observers. The earthbound fluid mechanics-dynamics community is joined in this challenge by an even less expected group, astrophysical planetary scientists. They are intrigued because space probes have shown strange and often very wildly turbulent mixed vapor/fluid atmospheres on other members of the solar system. The "eye" of Jupiter, for example, is a hurricane that has been going on for literally hundreds of years!

Awareness of the interconnectedness of air-ocean and gas-liquid phenomena has not, however, led to the abandonment of independent specialty professional societies within the geophysical sciences. Many of these specialty societies have separate professional journals, and read and cite papers in a somewhat inner-looking fashion. Moreover, for-profit publishers remain interested in marketing distinct titles to as many niches as can be discerned.

## SOURCES OF REVIEWS

Only a few specialties within the oceanic-atmospheric continuum have serials primarily devoted to reviews, and relatively few journals in general science or in general geophysics feature oceanic and atmospheric reviews regularly. Even the recounting of these meager sources is choppy.

The physical oceanography segment of the field is blessed with more reviews than most of its neighboring disciplines. The two leaders are the *Ocean Yearbook*, a hardbound with a fair amount of biological oceanography, handled by the University of Chicago Press for the International Oceanographic Institute, and *Progress in Oceanography*, a more heavily "physical" oceanography series, from Pergamon. The former has a mixture of state-of-the-art and installment reviews, the latter almost exclusively emphasizes lengthy state-of-the-art reviews. While it is worth the wait, the *Yearbook* habitually lags in production, averaging about 18 months between appearances. *Progress*, by contrast, regularly appears eight times a year as a softbound serial. These two are joined by something a bit more readable. Popular level oceanographic reviews, with both physical and life science aspects, can be found in *Oceanus* from the Woods Hole Oceanographic Institute. All three serials are strongly recommended for every collection in ocean and atmospheric sciences.

*Oceanography and Marine Biology* from Aberdeen University Press is a hardbound with extensive state-of-the-art essays, but is much more biological than the others in this group. It is optional for most geophysical collections.

The *Journal of Physical Oceanography* from the American Meteorological Society and the *Journal of Geophysical Research–Oceans* from the American Geophysical Union are leaders in this field, and mandatory for reasons of their excellent articles of original research. Neither, however, regularly features reviews.

The meteorological contingent has no purely dedicated review journals. The need for overviews is served partly by a popular journal which has some tutorial reviews, *Weatherwise* from Heldref, and partly by *Weather* from the (British) Royal Meteorological Society, which provides occasional, higher level state-of-the-art reviews. The American Meteorological Society publishes a wide variety of journals, but the "reviews" they contain are both sporadic and have a special character, fairly unique to meteorology's occupational concerns. *Monthly Weather Review* provides the best example of this situation with its penchant for extended weather histories and longer range verification studies. This means one can find papers summarizing the circulation patterns of a whole season, and perhaps a detailed comparison between what was predicted for a season and what actually happened. A somewhat more conventional type of review, akin to the installment plan review of technical progress over a given time, can be found in the *Bulletin of the American Meteorological Society*. The *Bulletin*'s somewhat informal progress reports typically deal with large scale, long-term, cooperative efforts to monitor the weather via land radar networks, or by an array of ocean buoys, or via a new weather satellite.

Very long-term weather studies from dozens to thousands of years are the essential grist of climatology. Once again, there are no specifically designated review journals, but given the long-term correlation and integration of records involved in any climatic studies of more modern times, many papers do have a review character. This is particularly true of the papers in *Climatic Change*, a Kluwer journal. An intermediate number of reviews are to be found in the leading British entry, *Wiley's International Journal of Climatology*, and the historically German, but increasingly international *Theoretical and Applied Climatology* from Springer. Perhaps unfortunately, the leading U.S. title, the prestigious *Journal of Climate* from the American Meteorological Society, has the fewest reviews overall. It is actually easier to find reviews dealing with climatological periods more than a few thousand years ago. *Quaternary Science Reviews* from Pergamon, while not strictly a climatological journal, has as many climatology reviews as most of the strictly climatological titles. "Quaternary" refers to the last two or three million years of earth history.

The atmospheric sciences contingent features reviews scattered throughout a number of their principal journals. This is particularly true of the European and/or for-profit publishing sectors. *Atmospheric Research*, a now largely English language Elsevier journal with a French background, and *Meteorology and Atmospheric Physics*, a Springer entry with a German academic history, are good examples. The *Journal of the Atmospheric Sciences*, the American Meteorological Society entry, has few reviews. *Advances in the Atmospheric Sciences*, an irregular hardbound Elsevier series, occasionally has a collection of reviews, but is generally a monographic series.

The leading source of state of the art surveys for the fluid dynamical modeling community is the *Annual Reviews of Fluid Mechanics*. Some extended tutorial surveys can be found in Cambridge University's *Journal of Fluid Mechanics*. It is not unusual for the highly mathematicized papers there to run thirty pages, and to involve a good deal more step-by-step discussion than is found in most other physics journals.

## SYMPOSIA AND THEME ISSUES

As with reviews, oceanic symposia also have few journals dedicated solely to them. Scattered appearances of proceedings are quite common, but the locations are not always consistent.

The leading international title is, however, the *ICES Marine Sciences Symposia* from the International Council for the Exploration of the Sea. Not surprisingly for a field that has substantial European involvement, it is Danish of origin, and still has some French language content. The American Society for Limnology and Oceanography holds annual workshops, and sometimes includes workshop papers within their flagship journal, *Limnology and Oceanography*. But at least partly because ASLO is a fairly small and modestly funded group, they have also published their collective works in Canadian journals, which are well supported, and in some American Geophysical Union vehicles, such as the *Journal of Geophysical Research–Oceans*.

The conference literature in meteorology is, much like that of oceanography, highly international. The global leader is the *Proceedings, World Meteorological Congress*, published by the World Meteorological Organization. The WMO is headquartered in Switzerland and serves as the the UN's vehicle for a broad array of multilingual publications in meteorology. The American Meteorological Society handles WMO publications within the U.S. Most collections will want the quadrennial WMO congress documents and the *Annual Reports*. The American Meteorological Society also publishes *Meteorological Monographs* on its own. While the title may suggest that most of these irregular issues are extended treatments by individual authors, they are in fact, frequently, theme issues or collections of symposia papers. They are also required in virtually all oceanic and atmospheric collections.

In more recent years, there has been a divison between those journals which stress man-made or other recent era climatic changes and those which stress changes over geologic time scales. Both recent and geologic categories of journals tend to have many symposia and theme issues. In the more "recent" category we find that *Climatic Change* from Kluwer, noted earlier for reviews, also features a substantial number of symposia. *Global and Planetary*

*Change* is its Elsevier competitor, and likewise features symposia. *Paleogeography, Paleoclimatology, and Paleoecology* from Elsevier perfectly describes in its title the interacting disciplines that help climatologists decide what planetary conditions were like thousands of years ago. Climatologists often seek help from paleontologists, geologists, and physical geographers in their decision making. Paleontologists look at the fossil record and geologists have an understanding of shifts in tectonic plates, while geographers trace events in the sedimentation of rivers or the rise of volcanos. Through the aid of these cognate scientists, climatologists can make sense of tropical plant traces in a currently cold climate or coral remains on mountaintops. Not surprisingly, many of the symposia that do appear in *Paleogeography, Paleoclimatology, and Paleoecology* are interdisciplinary.

Two journals devoted largely to glaciers and the cold regions occasionally publish symposia and are important adjuncts to climatological studies. These are *Boreas* from the Scandinavian publisher Universitetsforlaget, and the *Journal of Glaciology* from the International Glaciological Society. Not only are most glaciers tens of thousands of years old, and of intrinsic interest, but their ice often contains chemical clues to atmospheric makeup during precipitation events whose hallmarks are well-preserved in frozen layers. Was there acid rain 5,000 years ago? In what eras did there appear to be warmer temperatures or less rain? Climatologists drill through polar or glacial ice in much the same same way that geophysicists drill through the earth's crust, or botanists bore through the rings of ancient sequoias.

Symposia are plentiful in the atmospheric sector of atmospheric-oceanic studies. The American Geophysical Union frequently publishes symposia in the *Journal of Geophysical Research–Atmospheres* and in the *Journal of Geophysical Research–Space Physics*. While most collections will want both titles, the former deals more often with matter that more intimately affect weather and climate-related phenomena, the latter with long-range cosmic interactions. The leading for-profit competition to the AGU comes from three publishers. Symposia in *Boundary Layer Meteorology* from Kluwer cover atmospheric phenomena up to a kilometer. A greater height is often seen in symposia in Elsevier's *Dynamics of Oceans and At-*

*mospheres*, with the most flexible and extensive definition of factors that affect weather and climate used in symposia in Pergamon's *Journal of Atmospheric and Terrestrial Physics*.

## *METHODS*

The dominant methods serial in this area is clearly the *Journal of Atmospheric and Oceanic Technology*. This American Meteorological Society publication covers all the equipment and increasingly much of the software necessary for ground- and water-based observatories, and both balloon- and satellite-based sensing. Methods papers also appear in other meteorological journals. The journal that most of us would associate with meteorologists on television would be *Weather and Forecasting* from the AMS. Yet, there are other applications of weather and climate that stress practical concerns and technique. The *Journal of Applied Meteorology* from the AMS includes the weather as affecting crops, utilities, and city services. *Agricultural and Forest Meteorology* from Elsevier is a good companion. Soil moisture, structure, and fertility as affected by weather are dealt with in many journals of agronomy.

The technical reports series of many individual oceanographic institutes contain a great deal of reference data and descriptions of the experimental setups used to obtain them. Bulletins from the Woods Hole Oceanographic Institute and Scripps are among those more widely collected in the U.S.

The mathematically and computationally fluid dynamicist will find the *International Journal of Numerical Methods in Fluids* and *Computers and Fluids* from Pergamon essential, although as with much of the fluid literature, a great many chemical engineering papers will also be found. A mixed constituency will also be seen in the American Institute of Physics title *Physics of Fluids*. "Section A," available separately, has the greatest relevance to oceanic and atmospheric workers. The *Journal of Fluid Mechanics* from Cambridge University Press, mentioned earlier as a source of reviews carries mathematical methods papers regularly.

# Organic Chemistry

The phrase "organic chemistry" denotes the chemistry of carbon-containing compounds. Since compounds containing significant amounts of carbon are dominant in both living material and in many synthetic substances, it is not surprising that organic chemistry is arguably the first or second most important specialty in most academic departments of chemistry. (Biochemists now tend to outnumber organic chemists, except where the biochemists have their own department.) Organic chemistry is also key to much chemical engineering as well, particularly where medicines, plastics, and petroleum are the focus. There are many significant categories of organic compounds (e.g., heterocyclics) and some chemists categorize their interest by family of compounds. The majority of organic chemists, however, see themselves as one or more of the following. First, there are extractors and characterizers of organic compounds from raw materials (natural products chemists). Second, there are synthesizers of new organic organic compounds from scratch (synthetic organic chemists). Third are explainers of the structure and conditions for the transformation of organic compounds (physical organic chemists). It is arguable that synthetic chemists–the glamour group within this field–get their ideas of what to make artificially from the natural products community, and get their explanations for why given attempts to make it will or will not succeed from analyses done by the physical chemists.

Whatever their emphasis, organic chemists have been among the best served by special literature throughout history. There have been many important multivolume *Handbücher*, encyclopedias, dictio-

[Haworth co-indexing entry note]: "Organic Chemistry." Stankus, Tony. Co-published simultaneously in *The Serials Librarian* (The Haworth Press, Inc.) Vol. 27, No. 2/3, 1995, pp. 171-180; and: *Special Format Serials and Issues: Annual Review of . . . , Advances in . . . , Symposia on . . . , Methods in . . .* (ed: Tony Stankus) The Haworth Press, Inc., 1995, pp. 171-180. Single or multiple copies of this article are available from The Haworth Document Delivery Service [1-800-342-9678, 9:00 a.m. - 5:00 p.m. (EST)].

naries, and serially issued reference books, some dating back through the turn of the century. Most are known by the surnames of their earliest compilers or by a short list that includes their successors as well. *Beilstein, Houben/Weyl, Theilheimer, Heilbron, Fieser and Fieser, Harrison and Harrison/Wade/Smith* are among the many. Some of these works tend to rely on rather unique chemical structure schematic diagrams or flow charts to serve as abstracts or indices to literature published elsewhere–a system entirely appropriate to organic chemistry–but often have surprisingly little prose themselves. Since they are already well-explained in guides to the literature of chemistry, they get only selective and brief mentions here. This chapter will concentrate on works which provide their readers with more extensive background, discussion and procedural details within their own pages; at the same time they refer their readers to other sources.

## *REVIEWS IN ORGANIC CHEMISTRY APPEARING IN JOURNALS OF MORE GENERAL CHEMICAL INTEREST*

Reviews of organic chemistry rarely, if ever, appear in the major general science journals. This is partly because chemists, apart from biochemists, infrequently publish any kind of paper in non-chemistry journals. Moreover, there are many good outlets specializing in reviews of chemistry.

The most important source of reviews among general chemistry journals is *Angewandte Chemie–International Edition in English.* Indeed, this VCH publication is one of the last general interest chemistry journals to routinely allow reviews alongside regular articles and brief letters. It is an outstanding exception and belongs in virtually every chemistry library in America. The reviews in *Angewandte Chemie* are typically medium length and state-of-the-art although, as an important Continental publication, some life-and-times material is often included.

All the leading serials specifically devoted to reviews in general chemistry welcome papers in organic chemistry. Three of these sources are regularly-issued softbounds. The fourth is a somewhat irregularly issued hardbound.

The world leader is the American Chemical Society's *Chemical*

*Reviews*, a softbound bimonthly. The papers inside an issue are almost monstrously exhaustive, and generally encompass both historical and state-of-the-art aspects. Both the British and Germans have comparable publications with similarly extensive traditional reviews. The Royal Society of Chemistry publishes *Chemical Society Reviews*, with some life-and-times commentary in its pieces, although primarily state-of-the-art in intent. Springer, the German giant, publishes the hardbound *Current Topics in Chemistry*, a direct, albeit English-language, descendant of its *Fortschritte der Chemischen Forschung*.

The fourth significant journal, *Accounts of Chemical Research*, strongly favors minireviews. This slender monthly features state-of-the-art works. Although the tone is informal and focuses primarily on the author's own laboratory, these papers can be somewhat provocative.

The minimum assortment for small libraries should be *Chemical Reviews* and the *Accounts*. Both of the remaining reviews are highly valuable. A slight nod goes to *Chemical Society Reviews* over *Topics* owing to its greater regularity and predictability of price.

## SERIALS DEVOTED TO REVIEWS SPECIFICALLY IN ORGANIC CHEMISTRY

Journals covering all phases of organic chemistry, whether involving full-length papers or brief preliminary communications, rarely mix in review papers. There is a notable exception: *Tetrahedron*, a Pergamon entry that publishes full-length papers in organic chemistry, also accepts a significant number of reviews. These are termed "*Tetrahedron* Reports," and are available separately for those without a subscription to this leading journal.

Three hardbound review sources cover broad areas of organic chemistry. The first is a British publication favoring installment works, the *Annual Reports on the Progress of Chemistry: Section B; Organic Chemistry* from the Royal Society of Chemistry. The remaining two are American, and favor state-of-the-art surveys. These are *Organic Reaction Mechanisms*, as well as *Organic Reactions*, both from Wiley. The British entry offers the widest vista, with a relatively larger share of papers in the less popular, natural products and physical organic areas. The American entries, particularly *Organic Reactions*, have some bias for topics that are of principal interest to synthetic chemists. It would be hard to imagine not taking all three services, with *Organic Reactions* having the lead anywhere synthesis is done, and the *Annual Reports* being the best choice in a small collection with no clear emphasis.

## SOURCES OF MORE SPECIALIZED REVIEWS IN ORGANIC CHEMISTRY

Each of the major subspecialties within organic chemistry also has one or more special genre serials. Selection strategy should proceed on the presence or absence of these specialties in your user community.

The natural products area has the Royal Society of Chemistry's *Natural Products Reports*, a softbound bimonthly, and Springer's venerable *Fortschritte der Chemie Organischer Naturstoffe*, an irregular hardbound mercifully subtitled *Progress in the Chemistry of Organic Natural Products*. Despite the Teutonic main title, the bulk of its extensive state-of-the-art reviews are nowadays in English. The newer British title is a better first choice than this German entry, in smaller collections.

The physical organic area has Academic's *Advances in Physical Organic Chemistry*, a roughly annual hardbound. While the main approach in *Advances* is state-of-the-art, its editors explicitly insist that enough tutorial and life-and-times detail be included so as to enable a newcomer to the field to understand the background and motivation of the theme discussed. Wiley has a comparable hardbound series, *Progress in Physical Organic Chemistry*. It favors extensive state-of-the-art reviews, suitable largely for the most advanced readers. Unfortunately, the Wiley entry has had some exceptionally long pauses between the appearance of its valuable volumes, and this suggests a greater reliance on the Academic Press title in most collections.

The synthetic area has a prominent review serial (which has undergone a recent shift in format) and two other sources of strong reviews in journals that feature other types of articles as well. Formerly, the Royal Society of Chemistry published *General and*

*Synthetic Methods Specialist Periodical Reports.* It was a hard-bound featuring roughly annual installment reviews and clearly belonged in every library collection of any size. The RSC has now switched to a softbound bimonthly, *Contemporary Organic Synthesis*, while keeping its installment review nature (for some papers) and high quality (for seemingly all of them). The change was made partly to offset the problem of getting timely enough installments for each important area of organic synthesis ready all at once. These are now spread out over the year, and many more new themes can be taken up, whether or not they promise to be recurring. While the substantial merit of this serial is unchanged, it is not clear that the understandable price increase that accompanied the greater frequency will be greeted by librarians. It should remain a first choice for serious collections.

Reviews in two regular journals of organic synthesis, *Synthesis*, and its offspring for brief communications, *Synlett*, may have had some of their thunder stolen by the changes in the RSC's *Contemporary Organic Synthesis*. Nonetheless, both are largely English-language publications from Thieme, a reputable German scientific and medical publisher, and share a state-of-the-art approach. *Synthesis*, which generally features full-length papers, has the more formal and lengthier surveys, and terms them "Reviews." *Synlett*, by contrast, features minireviews, which it terms "Accounts." Their contrasting format lengths mirror the distinctions between the American Chemical Society's *Chemical Reviews* and its *Accounts of Chemical Research*. These Thieme products will continue to be of importance, and as they are readily taken for their original research, access to their reviews is likely to continue.

It is regrettable that two hardbound review series appear to be in abeyance. These were Wiley's *The Total Synthesis of Natural Products* edited by the redoubtable John ApSimon, and Elsevier's *Studies in Natural Products Chemistry*, from Atta-ur-Rahman. As a genre, they were in that gray area between encyclopedic schematic indexing/abstracting services and genuine reviews, but tended to have more readable prose sections than many of their peers. They also covered their special interest within organic chemistry very well and bridged many an interdisciplinary gap.

The finer levels of subspecialization in organic chemistry also support reviews, generally of the state-of-the-art school. Some of these publications are conceptually based, others concern categories of compounds. A leading example of a largely conceptual approach is found in *Topics in Stereochemistry*, a Wiley hardbound appearing somewhat irregularly. Stereochemistry is the study of the surprisingly sharp differences of behavior in a compound wrought by the subtle rearrangement in three dimensional space of some of its parts. While physical organic chemists make stereochemistry one of their major concerns, it is also important to natural products chemists who find mirror-twin compounds in nature, and to synthetic chemists who seek to make one spatial version of a compound without interference or contamination by what used to be called a "stereoisomer."

Yet another category of review serial in organic chemistry is based on a structural novelty. It stems from the propensity of carbon atoms to form rings. Such compounds are said to be cyclic. The most intriguing cyclics or rings have one or more of the carbon sites evacuated and an atom of nitrogen, oxygen, or some other non-carbon serving as a replacement, rendering them "heterocyclics." Both natural products and synthetic chemists tend to study these, and Academic fields a review serial to serve them, *Advances in Heterocyclic Chemistry*. Like most members of the Academic family, it features extensive, state-of-the-art reviews in a roughly annual hardbound format. It should be noted that two more regularly issued journals occasionally publish reviews. *Heterocycles*, handled by Elsevier for the Japanese Heterocyclic Society, has English language surveys alongside its largely brief communications format. The *Journal of Heterocyclic Chemistry*, from the HeteroCorporation, issues supplements called "Lectures in Heterocyclic Chemistry." These often include tutorial, and life-and-times reviews as well as the more common state-of-the-art approach.

## REVIEWS OF ORGANIC CHEMISTRY THAT ARE IMPORTANT TO NEIGHBORING DISCIPLINES

Installment reviews are common in three other organically related members of the Royal Society of Chemistry family. Their emphasis is primarily chemical, but their appeal includes other disciplines and industry. These include *Amino Acids and Peptides*, and two versions of *Carbohydrate Chemistry*, one subtitled *Part 1: Mono-Di-Tri-Saccharides and Their Derivatives*, the other, *Part 2: Macromolecules*. All three are *Specialist Periodical Reports* and roughly annual hardbounds. The first two titles are of special interest to biochemists: amino acids and peptides are the building blocks of proteins while the saccharides include many natural sugars. The third title has both biochemical and industrial interest: it deals with starches, gels, and biopolymers.

Another example of a review serial bridging both organic and biochemical communities is Academic's *Advances in Carbohydrate Chemistry and Biochemistry*. Its papers are generally of the extended state-of-the-art type.

The best review link between organic chemists and the pharmaceuticals industry is *Medicinal Research Reviews*, a softbound from Wiley. It has the strongest synthetic chemistry (as opposed to metabolic biology) slant among reviews in this area. The neighboring field of pharmacology is better served by more physiologically inclined journals. (See the chapters on physiology and pharmacology.)

Review journals bridge the industrial polymer and organic chemistry communities. One example is a separate journal for reviews split off from an originally multifunctional journal: the *Journal of Macromolecular Science. Part C. Reviews in Macromolecular Chemistry and Physics*, from Dekker. An entirely independent journal, *Progress in Polymer Science* from Pergamon is its leading competitor. Both are softbounds, the first quarterly, the second bimonthly. Interestingly, because readers with an interest in polymers come from a variety of technical backgrounds, reviews in both these serials tend to have a substantial tutorial component as the authors seek to get their diversified audiences up to the same speed before going deeper into the topic.

## SYMPOSIA AND THEME ISSUES IN ORGANIC CHEMISTRY

One major softbound journal devoted to all fields of chemistry frequently features symposia in organic chemistry. That is *Pure and*

*Applied Chemistry*, a publication of the International Union for *Pure and Applied Chemistry* handled by Blackwell. This is especially strong in European synthetic work, although one of its other specialties, the publication of standardized names for compounds and of rules for formulating those names, is critical to all types of organic chemists.

The American Chemical Society has a partial counterpart to *Pure and Applied Chemistry*, but it differs in format, frequency, and amount devoted to organic chemistry. The *ACS Symposium Series* encompasses up to twenty hardbound volumes annually, and covers a very wide range of topics. Its method of compilation is a hybrid of the symposia and the theme issue. While most of the papers are the result of live presentations, some later revision of the text, and even some reporter-summarized material can be included. Interestingly, related papers from different national meetings can be merged into a single thematic volume. Camera-ready-copy is used to get these volumes to press sooner, although some volumes appear mostly typeset. In recent years, industrial aspects of chemistry seem more stressed than academic areas. Nonetheless, the series is well worth monitoring for selective purchase of individual volumes of interest to organic chemists.

While a number of journals specifically devoted to organic chemistry occasionally feature symposia, *Tetrahedron* consistently features a number every year. In a series entitled "*Tetrahedron* Symposia in Print," both collections of papers from "live" symposia and thematically oriented collections of separately submitted papers appear, representing some of the best Continental and Commonwealth work.

The appearance of symposia and theme issues in the various subspecialties within organic chemistry is also erratic. One notable exception is Wiley's *Journal of Polymer Science: Polymer Symposia Edition*, an irregular hardbound.

## METHODS SERIALS IN ORGANIC CHEMISTRY

Very few disciplines have the rich array of *Handbuch* type methods works possessed by organic chemists. Because organic synthesis, the dominant specialty, is the making of new compounds (or the making of old compounds in new ways), encyclopedic recipe books are legion. Many are gigantic and are rarely handled as serials so much as quasi-indexing-abstracting tools or reference encyclopedias. Nonetheless, at least three should be mentioned here briefly, with a fourth with greater "serials character" discussed more thoroughly. The most comprehensive is of, course, *Beilsteins Handbuch der Organischen Chemie*, a series distributed by Springer. Deeply respected, somewhat arcane of organization and indexing, and exceptionally expensive, it is one of the prototypical "encyclopedias-without-end." It has a British counterpart with a great deal more prose, *Rodd's Chemistry of Carbon Compounds*, handled by Elsevier. (*Beilstein* has prose, but is heavily into brief facts, physical data, and cross-referencing.) Finally, there is *Theilheimer's Synthetic Methods of Organic Chemistry*, distributed by Karger. Each of these works is hardbound. Each attempts to have a subject section-by-section or subject volume-by-volume approach, and is updated in its print versions through new volumes or editions that maintain that scheme, even if it involves a bit of uneven growth among the various classified parts. It is not surprising that many series in this vein are rapidly developing parallel on-line versions, which permit much easier searching. Some are full-text and it is not clear that the print versions will continue in the long run.

The most thriving serial that serves a methods approach works on a much simpler premise. *Organic Syntheses* is a roughly annual hardbound which provides completely clear procedures for the making of particularly novel or useful compounds. Although most papers are rather brief, instrumentation and starting materials are unambiguously inventoried and detailed. Notes of proven yields, contaminants that may occur, and any hazards involved are easy to find. Most importantly, the authors include not only those who have originally proposed and initially executed the synthesis, but the professionals at other institutions who have repeated the procedure, and found it trustworthy. In the most recent volumes a number of innovations have occurred. First, camera-ready-copy is being used as both a time and money saver, with a softbound preliminary version being sent out to individual subscribers, and a finished hardbound with indexing available for libraries. Second, a list of proposed syntheses "in search of independent checkers" is posted so as to more quickly confirm the claims of new and useful procedures. It should be noted that both old and new versions of *Organic Syntheses* are also available in handy, relatively inexpensive cumulations. Newer editions typically cover five-year spans.

# Physiology and Selected Areas of Internal Medicine

Physiology is the evaluation of bodily function. It measures. It looks for explanations of good and bad performance. It examines evidence as obvious as gross deterioration in a sizeable body part right down to something as subtle as a defect in a cell's ability to process a single protein. While fundamental, molecular physiologists suggest that the truth always lies closer to the cellular end, the working physiologists we call physicians still tend to treat whole patients and specialize by major organ system.

Not all organ systems are created equal, however, in terms of the number of current scientific or clinical adherents. As a practical matter, cardiologists dominate the wards (clinical literature) while endocrinologists seem to rule the labs (journals of basic science). This weighting is reflected in the number and capaciousness of serials in these areas, and in the need for freestanding review, symposia, and methods sources. Indeed the number and special nature of neuroscience journals requires their treatment in an entirely separate chapter.

While schools of medicine and pharmacology are probably the largest sponsors of physiological research today, at least two other groups ought to be noted. Like the medical contingent, the first of the alternative groups is primarily concerned with humans: the applied physiologists. They stress the energetics and biomechanics demanded by exercise and physically vigorous occupations. The

[Haworth co-indexing entry note]: "Physiology and Selected Areas of Internal Medicine." Stankus, Tony. Co-published simultaneously in *The Serials Librarian* (The Haworth Press, Inc.) Vol. 27, No. 2/3, 1995, pp. 181-198; and: *Special Format Serials and Issues: Annual Review of . . . , Advances in . . . , Symposia on . . . , Methods in . . .* (ed: Tony Stankus) The Haworth Press, Inc., 1995, pp. 181-198. Single or multiple copies of this article are available from The Haworth Document Delivery Service [1-800-342-9678, 9:00 a.m. - 5:00 p.m. (EST)].

interactions of heart, lung, and skeletal muscle dominate their agenda. This contingent has been extraordinarily well-funded in the former communist bloc under the guise of "sports science." In the U.S., there is growing interest in this field from what used to be called the "physical education" community. It should be noted however, that "sports medicine" in the United States tends to include a good deal more orthopedic and podiatric surgery than is seen in the European context. This is reflected in a somewhat less purely physiological tone in American journals in the field. To a degree, Europeans stress enhancement of performance, while Americans stress repair of injuries.

The second group of alternative physiologists tends to work with many types of animals, and has less concern as to whether or not the performance of those animals illuminates the human experience. These are the comparative or adaptational physiologists. They also study function and performance, but with a different slant. They wish to understand how features of a given animal help it survive environmental stresses, especially those that humans rarely face to these extremes: how whales hold their breath for hours; how camels last so long without a drink; how a monkey swings its whole body weight by its arms through the trees.

On the whole physiologists who seek to understand humans, at the molecular, cellular, and organ system levels, tend to outnumber comparative physiologists. This chapter could therefore be easily dominated by mention of over 100 general purpose journals of clinical internal medicine, because physiology is their core concern. But as a practical matter, this chapter will stress only those general clinical journals that tend to be of such high standing that an overwhelming segment of the medical community will need them. Organ systems journals will also be treated selectively. As we've noted above, many doctors specialize by type of organ system. They have established a network of organ system journals that far exceeds those few founded by comparative physiologists. Fortunately for comparative physiologists, some of these largely clinical organ system journals entertain reviews, conferences, and methods papers dealing with nonhuman subjects.

## REVIEWS OF HUMAN PHYSIOLOGY
## AND MODEL SYSTEMS FOR HUMAN PHYSIOLOGY

Major multiscience journals such as *Science* and *Nature* will occasionally carry reviews dealing with human cellular physiology or with some unique adaptational mechanism in freely roaming animals. *FASEB Journal* carries them somewhat more frequently, and its reviews are now cited at an equally high rate. However, the bulk of today's physiology surveys appear in reading aimed more or less exclusively at physiologists.

Three series should be in all collections. The first is *Physiological Reviews* from the American Physiological Society. A bimonthly softbound, it features some of the longest, and most comprehensive papers in the field. It is not unusual for a typical state-of-the-art survey to run over 50 pages with over 500 references nicely integrated. Its most serious competiton is from the not-for-profit Annual Reviews, Inc. Their *Annual Review of Physiology* offers intermediate-length papers, usually between a dozen and twenty pages, with the customary life-and-times biographical introduction followed by a dozen or so state-of-the-art entries. *News in Physiological Sciences* is a somewhat lighter, more tutorial-and-minireview-oriented vehicle that also contains, as its title suggests, professional society news. Sponsored by the American Physiological Society and the International Union of Physiological Sciences, this bimonthly is almost as much a bargain as the *Annual Reviews.* In a most happy coincidence of good values, few institutions will have to make hard financial choices between these leaders, and will have all three.

A fourth choice is less carefree. Springer has a longstanding irregular, hardbound series, *Reviews of Physiology, Biochemistry, and Pharmacology.* While its title indicates the essential intertwining of these fields, and the series has had some particularly heavily cited papers from the Continental European community from time-to-time, it has not been a consistent performer. Given that in a typical year of two or three numbers it costs at least twice as much as its competition, it might be reserved for the largest medical and pharmacological collections.

While the bulk of general interest review reporting is handled by the four review sources just mentioned, irregularly appearing reviews are also a feature of a fairly small number of journals of general physiology. These include two journals devoted primarily to regular research articles. Full-length review papers are to be found in *Experimental Physiology* from Cambridge University Press. Minireviews are not uncommon in the *Proceedings of the Society of Experimental Biology and Medicine*, the vehicle of a venerable New York City-based group, handled by Williams and Wilkins. These are both journals of intermediate standing, but this review-serving function might enhance decisions to add or retain them in collections.

## JOURNALS OF CLINICAL MEDICINE
## AS REVIEW SOURCES IN PHYSIOLOGY

Clinical physiology is well covered by occasionally appearing reviews in an army of journals of internal medicine. Few journals of general clinical practice or investigative internal medicine are entirely without reviews during the course of the year, although their timing and number in any given year are not always predictable.

There are major distinctions between reviews in journals specifically devoted to physiology surveys, and these important but irregular items in journals of general medicine. Reviews in journals of clinical medicine aim for "consensus." While the lengthy give-and-take of some of the state-of-the art papers that dominates the review journals of physiology noted above is not absolutely excluded in clinical journals, there is a greater sense of finality and resolution. Despite the fact that these clinical journal reviews are often shorter than research journal reviews, many of these clinical consensus reviews feature a large panel of authors, something that is rarely seen in reviews in basic sciences. The idea is often one of lending as much weight as possible to the conclusions of the review.

Another related "pro-consensus" development in a number of clinical journals is the recapitulation minireview or endorsing editorial. Here the editors summarize and reinforce the main points of a number of original research papers, often those appearing in the same issue, with some allusion to similar papers in reputable competitors. This need for safety in numbers, both among the original authors, and among the members of the editorial board issuing the endorsement, is clearly related to a hope for standardization of clinical practices. Working physicians seek to be supplied with information that they can use not only to treat patients, but to defend themselves against liability in the event of an unfortunate outcome. The defense of a "consensus of opinion in a leading journal" is powerful. It offers reassurance to working physicians who cannot keep up with every little experimental advance. Working physicians can readily admit in court, and before peer review panels in hospitals, that there are dozens of possible findings that *might* benefit a patient that could have been overlooked in their reading, but that it may in any case, have been unwise to apply them to the patient under question until a consensus has been reached as to their efficacy and safety. Those physicians may justly argue that they were waiting for such a consensus to be reported in a number of star-quality journals.

The leading journals for such clinical reviews are the *New England Journal of Medicine* from the Massachusetts Medical Society, the *Annals of Internal Medicine* from the American College of Physicians, the *Archives of Internal Medicine* from the American Medical Association, the *American Journal of Medicine* from Cahners and the *American Journal of Medical Sciences* from Lippincott. Pediatrics is covered by a number of titles, one of which is famous for its endorsing minireviews. "The Editorial Board Speaks" is a regular feature of the AMA's *Archives of Pediatrics and Adolescent Medicine*. Fortunately, virtually every medical and pharmaceutical library, and many in the more basic sciences, is likely to have these several inexpensive titles on their shelves already. It should be stressed that there are many other excellent journals of medicine, *Lancet* and the *Journal of Experimental Medicine* come to mind, that are required reading for most physicians, but do not feature as many consensus reviews.

Consensus reviews are not the only kind of importance to medicine. The *Journal of the American Medical Association* is the leading example of a publisher of "installment reviews." In its annual "Contempo" issue, specially commissioned experts cover more than twenty areas of medicine. Its most significant competition among American audiences for this service lies in the *Annual Re-*

*view of Medicine,* which features a smaller and nonrecurring list of topical reviews, largely in state-of-the-art style.

Given that many clinical journals serve as organs of various societies, it is not unusual to find either awards lectures or scientific speeches by organizational leaders. The *Journal of Clinical Investigation,* which the Rockefeller University Press handles for the Society of Clinical Investigation, features an agenda-setting address which tends to be a kind of personalized "minireview" of developments important to its president, as well as "Perspectives," a more conventional if still somewhat informal review, in which either some intellectual speculation or historical allusion is allowed. Likewise, the *Canadian Journal of Physiology and Pharmacology* from that country's National Research Council features the Borden Award Lectures. Most of these combine a life-and-times introduction with a minireview of the work for which the award is being given: a standard formula for many honors addresses.

## REVIEWS IN APPLIED AND SPORTS PHYSIOLOGY

The applied, exercise, and ocupational physiology segment is served by an exceptionally regular series of "Brief Reviews" in the *Journal of Applied Physiology* from the American Physiological Society. More occassionally the *JAP* will feature a "Milestones in Physiology" reprint with a life-and-times commentary. *Medicine and Science in Sports and Exercise* from Williams and Wilkins features an annual "Memorial Lecture Series" which follows along the lines of an awards lecture.

## REVIEWS FOR COMPARATIVE PHYSIOLOGISTS

Adaptational physiology commands a large share among the lengthy state-of-the-art surveys in the *Quarterly Review of Biology,* a journal which the University of Chicago Press handles on behalf of the State University of New York at Stony Brook. Lengthy physiological reviews also do well in the *Biological Reviews of the Cambridge Philosophical Society,* the *Quarterly's* British peer. *Zoologische Jahrbücher–Abteilung für Allgemeine Zoologie und Physiologie der*

*Tiere* is the Continental European counterpart of the two previous, widely held English-language titles. Although it has tremendous historical importance to the entire review journal genre, it still features many foreign language articles and tends to be more expensive. It is recommended only for doctoral collections.

While there are well over a dozen significant general journals of zoology, only a few feature comparative physiology reviews. Two important journals feature them intermittently, one routinely.

There are two to four important "Invited Reviews" annually in the University of Chicago's *Physiological Zoology*, actually quite a feat given that journal's slender page count. Most of these are full-length and state-of-the-art. While it is sometimes criticized for treating only the "higher" order medical lab animals, important adaptational reviews can still be found in the *American Journal* of *Physiology: Regulatory, Integrative, and Comparative*. These reviews are occasional. There are one or two "honorary" reviews, usually tied in with the receipt of some distinction, and containing both life-and-times and state-of-the-art aspects; and two or three "Invited Reviews" of substantial length, almost always state-of-the-art surveys. By contrast, "minireviews" dealing with a very wide variety of animals are extremely frequent (20-30 annually) in Pergamon's *Comparative Biochemistry and Physiology*, one of the most voluminous journals in the field. *Physiological Zoology* should be in virtually every undergraduate collection in America, most medium to large collections will also want *CBP*, despite its significant costs. Comparative physiologists working in medical centers are the most likely audience for the reviews in *AJP*.

Journals more narrowly devoted to given categories of animals: birds, mammals, reptiles and amphibians, and the like, carry review papers dealing with their subject's adaptational physiology from time to time. As a rule, however, these journals tend to stress evolutionary classification, or behavior and habitat more than physiology. One important exception is the literature of the insects and their kin. The inexpensive *Annual Review of Entomology* from the Annual Reviews, Inc. and the more expensive, but also more focused *Advances in Insect Physiology*, an irregular hardbound from Academic, belong in any collection that studies invertebrate functioning.

## REVIEWS OF PHYSIOLOGICAL SPECIALTIES AND ORGANS SYSTEMS

### Endocrinology Including Diabetes and Sex Hormones

Endocrinologists seem to have the most extensive and best organized review network among the specialties. Three major services compete. *Endocrine Reviews* from the U.S.-based Endocrine Society is a softbound quarterly. *Recent Progress in Hormone Research* is a hardbound annual from Academic Press. While the first wins in citations, the second is also sound, and ironically for a for-profit publication, less expensive. Both favor very lengthy reviews for the involved researcher. The minireviews niche, and the winner of the readability contest, however, is Elsevier's *Trends in Endocrinology and Metabolism.* While it is the most expensive of the group, it is also the most readily accessible to the advanced undergraduate through its tutorials. It also contains highly interesting "Endocrine Rounds," clinical reviews for the working physician.

The endocrine network also includes a plethora of occasional reviews in journals primarily devoted to reports of original research. The leading journal, *Endocrinology,* from the leading professional group, the Endocrine Society, features life-and-times reviews as part of its "Remembrance Project." Two of its partner journals, *Molecular Endocrinology* and the *Journal of Clinical Endocrinology and Metabolism,* feature minireviews, the latter frequently mentioning diabetes. The less clinical, more fundamental American Physiological Society, issues a special section for hormone researchers: the *American Journal of Physiology: Endocrinology and Metabolism.* This section features occasional invited reviews (generally full-length and state-of-the-art), editorial reviews (generally "mini" and consensus-seeking), and awards and honors lectures (a fair amount of life-and-times detail). The less-heralded, U.S.-based *Endocrine Research,* from Dekker, has lengthier surveys than most of these other American journals, but they appear to have limited impact.

The British counter this large group of American review sources with a wide range of overview material in their flagship *Journal of Endocrinology* that has "Brief Commentaries," minireviews, and formal, full state-of-the-art reviews. "Commentary," a kind of editorial minireview, is common in Blackwell's *Clinical Endocrinology*, a good applied companion to the more fundamental *Journal.*

Elsevier's titanic *Molecular and Cellular Endocrinology*, a competitor of the U.S. Endocrine Society's *Molecular Endocrinology* and the U.K.'s *Journal of Molecular Endocrinology*, leads a largely Continental European contingent of authors with its feature "At the Cutting Edge," an intermittent series of critical and speculative minireviews. Its sternest competition on the Continent has come from Rhodos Press's *Acta Endocrinologica*, a Danish-based journal which features minireviews in its regular sequence of issues as well as special supplements with extended state-of-the-art surveys. This is not to discount either the minireviews in Thieme's *Hormone and Metabolic Research* or the the full-length surveys in Kurtis's *Journal of Endocrinological Investigation.*

Since most American libraries will have at least the first three U.S. titles as a matter of course, selection decisions among the remainder will focus on sorting out the British and Europeans. Since the provision of reviews is but one of several important factors, it cannot be decisive on its own. But as a practical matter, the presence of reviews strengthens the already economically and professionally strong case for both the *Journal of Endocrinology* and *Acta Endocrinologica*. It might make the considerable cost of *Molecular and Cellular Endocrinology* more tolerable. If the Elsevier entry is still financially unmanageable, then an assortment from among the remainder will approximate its value as a frequent review source at less cost.

It should be noted that two subspecialties tend to be intimately connected with hormone function. On the metabolic side, diabetes is the most common concern and most clinical collections will need access to the important but somewhat infrequent reviews in *Diabetes* (state-of-the-art) and *Diabetes Care* (tutorial) from the American Diabetes Association. The longest overviews in the field are found in Wiley's British-based *Diabetes-Metabolism Reviews*, which is recommended for medium-sized collections. *Diabetolog-*

*ica* from Springer has the best reviews from the Continental European contingent, and belongs in medical schools and tertiary care centers.

The other endocrine specialty of note is reproduction. While a plethora of andrological, gynecological, obstetric, and perinatal journals occasionally feature reviews, the best linkage between hormonal aspects and reproduction is found in the *Oxford Reviews in Reproductive Biology*, an irregular hardbound. It is recommended for both clinical and basic research collections.

### Heart and Circulatory

Because of the status of coronary disease as the number one killer of males in developed countries, the heart and circulatory system dominate as topics in most of the reviews in journals of general clinical medicine. Reviews there have exceptionally high "consensus" value. Yet this does not preclude the presence of other valuable surveys in four review journals specifically devoted to cardiology and vascular medicine, as well as occasional reviews in journals primarily intended for articles of original research and practice in coronary care.

*Modern Concepts in Cardiovascular Disease* is the current leader among the review sources. This American Heart Association publication is a unique slim softbound, devoted to a single tutorial review in each edition, largely intended for working clinicians. It is highly recommended, and a bargain to boot. It is not clear, however, whether or not *Modern Concepts* will be superseded by a brand new entry from the AHA, *Heart Disease and Stroke: A Journal for Primary Care Physicians*. This 1992 entry features papers that are fundamentally all invited review articles, although only the longest ones are labelled as such. There is a strong tutorial and consensus-seeking nature to most of the pieces. It certainly appears that there will be some duplication of function if both of these AHA titles continue.

Elsevier has recently entered the competition with yet another eminently readable *Trends* entry: *Trends in Cardiovascular Medicine*. It is more frequent, research-oriented, and cosmopolitan than its AHA competitors, with more of its minireviews referring to ongoing controversies. It is nonetheless a good companion to *Mod-*

*ern Concepts* and its new in-house competitor, *Heart Disease and Stroke*, for somewhat larger, better-budgeted collections.

The longer review is the staple of *Perspectives in Cardiovascular Research*, an irregular hardbound that sometimes has a review format, and sometimes features symposia. Despite the fact that it is senior to the *Trends* series, it has not made a deep and abiding impact. It is largely an item for major medical centers with comprehensive collections.

The American Heart Association also publishes several journals that primarily report original research in cardiovascular subspecialties. A number of these have occasional reviews. *Circulation* is arguably the most prominent for its wide spectrum of reviews under the categories of the "Research Advance Series" (state-of-the-art), "Special Reports" (clinical consensus), and "Clinical Progress" (ongoing trials, often in installment format). *Circulation Research* is *Circulation's* companion for more fundamental work. It has more animal studies and fewer clinical ones. Its reviews are also much more occasional. Closely behind these AHA publications are a number of other U.S. competitors, most notably the *American Heart Journal*. The *AHJ*, handled by Mosby, primarily features "Clinical Reviews," which are typically full-length and stress historical background leading to consensus on new treatments. A more fundamental research approach is found in the occasional reviews in the *American Journal of Physiology: Heart and Circulatory* from the American Physiological Society. Here the format is more mixed than the *American Heart Journal*, and reviews are more frequent than in *Circulation Research*. In the *AJP–Heart and Circulatory*, "Invited Reviews" are somewhat lengthy and stress state-of-the-art. "Editorial Reviews" are briefer and consensus-seeking, although as this is not a clinical journal, the goal is endorsement of a theoretical concept more than of some practical treatment. Finally, "Awards and Honors Lectures" include a good deal of introductory life-and-times detail along with a review that speaks to the current research emphasis of the recipient.

Selection decisions from among all these review choices might be made on an "intensely clinical" vs. "less clinical" orientation. The former would be better served by the reviews in *Circulation* and in the *American Heart Journal*; the latter by *Circulation Research* and the *American Journal of Physiology: Heart and Circulatory.*

### Pulmonary

While a good deal of healthy lung capacity and gas exchange work is covered by journals of applied, occupational, and sports physiology, reviews dealing with cellular levels of lung organization or with nonhuman subjects or with diseases of the lung can be found in a small but important cluster of journals that primarily feature original research articles. Minirevieviews can be found in *Experimental Lung Research*, from Hemisphere. Most are clinical in intent. Diseased human lungs are also the grist of review features entitled "Editorial," "State of the Art," "Pulmonary Perspective," and "Clinical Commentary," in the American Thoracic Society's *American Review of Respiratory Disease*. It should be noted that despite its "Review" title, and its plethora of largely consensus minireviews, this is not solely an organ for reviews. *Progress in Respiration Research* from Karger is, unlike its two regularly issued, softbound competitors, an irregular hardbound. Its reviews are the longest in pulmonary studies, although some volumes are symposia, with others essentially monographs. It shares an emphasis on lung pathology with its competitors, however.

The leader for reviews at the micro level, and the title with the most animal work is the *American Journal of Physiology: Lung Cellular and Molecular Physiology*. It follows the standard American Physiological Society format with a mix of frequent state-of-the-art, full-length reviews, and perhaps a single awards lecture with life-and-times and minireview aspects. In small collections, the *American Review* and the *American Journal* are clearly to be preferred for both cost and importance.

### The Gut

The digestive tract is less endowed with reviews than most other organ systems. A substantial number of the reviews deal with infectious diseases resulting from ingestions of microbes or parasites. Inborn metabolic diseases are actually fairly rare in the stomach, excepting for certain food intolerances.

Reviews are roughly monthly in *Gastroenterology*, a title which Elsevier handles for the American Gastroenterological Association. They are slightly rarer in the *American Journal of Gastoenterology* from the U.S.-based National Gastroenterological Association, and in *Digestive Diseases and Sciences* from Plenum.

*Hepatology* from Williams and Wilkins and *Diseases of the Colon and Rectum* from Lippincott are two of the more important subspecialty sources of occasional reviews from American doctors. *Gut* from the British Medical Association may add some non-American clinical review coverage.

The leader in the more basic research of the GI tract is the *American Journal of Physiology: Gastrointestinal and Liver Physiology*. It has the usual assortment of state-of-the-art invited reviews and the rarer awards life-and-times review. College collections would do well enough with the *American Journal*. Clinical collections will prefer the three more clinical U.S. titles. Major medical centers will need all the subspecialty titles as well.

### Fluid Balance and Elimination

The kidneys and bladder have a role beyond mere waste elimination. They serve as regulators of fluid and mineral salt balances that affect the heart and circulatory system as well. Moreover, the kidney has intimate connections both of body geography and biochemical functioning with parts of the endocrine system. Nonetheless, there are no serials exclusively devoted to fluid excretory survey papers. The clinical leader for reviews is the *Journal of Urology* which Williams and Wilkins handles. The stress there is overwhelming on obstructive diseases of males such as occur in prostate atrophy and cancer, or through infection. A somewhat better mix of occasional physiological reviews can be found in the *American Journal of Kidney Diseases*, a title that Saunders handles for the National Kidney Foundation.

The very best mix of reviews for the basic and comparative physiologist, however, is found in *Kidney International*, a Springer title, primarily for original research. Although it is more expensive than the ubiquitous American Physiological Society entry, the *American Journal of Physiology: Renal, Fluid, and Electrolyte Physiology*, both are recommended for even the smallest basic science collections for good coverage. In clinical settings, one should take the Williams and Wilkins and Saunders entries instead.

*Hypertension* from the American Heart Association may seem to be a surprising review source recommendation here, excepting that the most frequent cause of kidney failure is prolonged untreated high blood pressure, the flip side of the fact that fluid and electrolyte imbalances are one of the causes of high blood pressure.

## SYMPOSIA AND THEME ISSUES IN PHYSIOLOGY AND RELATED AREAS OF INTERNAL MEDICINE

Two firms dominate the theme and symposia issue trade in medically-related physiology: Saunders, and Grune and Stratton. Saunders features an extended hardbound series with members typically entitled *Clinics in . . .* Grune and Stratton use a generally quarterly softcover format to provide the same service with *Seminars in . . .* These distinctions of format and schedule are not absolute. Other firms market titles with similar introductory phrases and occasionally use each other's characteristic "lead-in," and there has been some switching back and forth of formats between irregular hardbounds and regular softbounds. Whatever their schedule, publisher or format, most of these following series feature theme issues rather than live symposia proceedings. Many of the component essays are tutorials, which may account for their relatively poor ranking as sources of citations in research journals. They are, nonetheless, highly instructive reading for busy practitioners and belong in any collection that matches the topic of the specialty under discussion.

Recommended series include *Clinics in Endocrinology and Metabolism* (Saunders) and *Bailliere's Clinical Endocrinology and Metabolism* (a British counterpart). Fertility and sterility experts will want *Seminars in Reproductive Endocrinology* (Thieme-Stratton). Heart and pulmonary work is covered by *Clinics in Chest Medicine* (Saunders) and *Seminars in Respiratory Medicine* (Stratton-Intercontinental). There are *Gastroenterological Clinics of North America* (Saunders) and *Bailliere's Clinical Gastroenterology*. Grune and Stratton features *Seminars in Nephrology*, Saunders counters partly with *Urologic Clinics of North America*.

Live symposia are common in journals of nonclinical, general physiology, as well as those of some organic systems. Curiously, some conference issues in the more academic journals are eclectic. They feature live symposia papers that have no tight, collective theme beyond being generally physiological, just a common location and conference sponsor. (This is seen with the regional conference issues of the otherwise extremely logically organized *Journal of Physiology* from Cambridge University Press.)

Among the endocrinologists, two journals seem to have more full-text symposia papers than their competition. These are *Hormone Research* from Karger, and the *Journal of Inherited Metabolic Diseases* from Kluwer.

The heart and circulatory system is served by symposia in the *American Journal of Cardiology* from Cahners, and the the *American Heart Journal* from Mosby. A Continental perspective is found in regular symposia supplements accompanying *Basic Research in Cardiology*, a Steinkopf publication. Hypertension symposia are frequent in a special *American Society of Hypertension: Symposium Series* and in frequent symposium supplements to a British source, the *Journal of Hypertension* from Current Science, UK. Symposia supplements are also an important feature of the *American Review of Respiratory Diseases*. The *Scandinavian Journal of Gastroenterology* from Universitatsforlaget always features at least one symposium supplement annually. The liver generates the most subspecialty symposia of any GI organ: the "Postgraduate Tutorials and Conferences" within Mosby"s *Hepatology,* and the "Symposia" within Thieme's *Hepato-Gastroenterology* are leading examples.

In the cases of American and British journals, the presence of symposia is a confirming factor for journals that are already prominent for their original research papers or reviews, and are therefore already likely to be selected. With some expensive Continental journals, symposia service can push a marginal title into a collection, particularly in tertiary referral hospitals and in medical school collections.

Symposia and theme issues are very important to four outstanding journals serving comparative physiologists. *American Zoologist*, while not solely devoted to physiology, is the premier theme/symposia journal of the field, and is the flagship title of the American Society of Zoologists. It belongs in every collection.

Close behind it are roughly semiannual conference supplements in the *Journal of Experimental Zoology*, a Wiley-Liss publication issued on behalf of the Section of Comparative Physiology of the American Society of Zoology. These papers are indeed the product of in-person presentations, but by editorial rule, all are submitted for subsequent refereeing by an after-the-meeting panel before appearing in a somewhat more polished form. Of equal stature are the ironically named supplementary "review volumes" of the equally ironically named *Journal of Experimental Biology*. These reviews are in fact symposia-in-print, and the biology discussed involves exclusively the animal kingdom. It is true that the individual contributions within these symposia tend to be review-like in the sense that they are formal, lengthy, and frequently involve extensive historical discussions of physiolgical concepts. A bonus with the *JEB* is its hardbound format and low cost owing to its not-for-profit British publisher, the Company of Biologists. The fourth member of the symposia team is notably more expensive than its peers, but already a strong contender for collection inclusion because of its strength in "minireviews." *Comparative Biochemistry and Physiology* from Pergamon frequently features live symposia papers, and does so with a greater and more exotic variety of location of species than its peers.

## METHODS IN PHYSIOLOGY

Classically, two objects were key to physiological experimentation. First, one needed a suitable animal or lab-sustained organ system or tissue. Second, one needed a measuring instrument for the activity under evaluation. Today, a statistical, mathematical, or computer-based guide to make sense of all the measurements seems just as necessary. Contemporary methods literature caters to all three concerns.

The principal journals dealing with the proper selection, care, and maintenance of intact animals are *Laboratory Animal Science* from the American Association for Laboratory Animal Science; a British counterpart, *Laboratory Science* from Laboratory Animals, Ltd.; and certain animal-specific vehicles, most notably the *Journal of Medical Primatology* from Karger, a title dealing largely with ape-like lab animals. Most collections that have very substantial and varied animal populations will also take one or more of the major veterinary journals. The *Journal of the American Veterinary Medical Association* and its more research-oriented companion title, the *American Journal of Veterinary Research* represent a good start.

The leading journals emphasizing instrumentation and measurement are largely human-oriented, and contain both a British and an American pair. It should be noted that alongside some monitoring and measuring papers, almost all the titles tend to have papers on delivering therapeutic beams or rays to destroy diseased tissue.

The U.K. contingent is co-sponsored by a number of Continental organizations. The paired journals consist of *Clinical Physics and Physiological Measurement* and *Physics in Medicine and Biology* from the Institute of Physical Sciences in Medicine, a subdivision of the Institute of Physics. While the latter title is senior of reputation and impact factor, the first deals more pertinently with physiological performance measurement as opposed to various radioactive therapies.

The pair of U.S. leaders are the *Medical Physics* from the American Institute of Physics and the *IEEE Transactions on Biomedical Engineering*. Unsurprisingly, the last title is the most equipment-focused and even includes the design of prosthetic devices. Despite this engineering tone, however, the *Transactions* actually includes more papers on physiological modelling than does *Medical Physics*, which has a greater diagnostic and therapeutic beam focus. In small collections, particularly outside of hospital settings, the *Transactions* is to be preferred.

Given categories of instrument also generate their own journals. For much of this century, the use of radio-opaque dyes and radioactive tracers has served to make the x-ray and its latter day enhancement, the CAT scan, important tools in physiological function testing. Radiological journals that cover x-rays and CAT scans were therefore more important to clinical physiology methods collections than might have been expected. However, the advent of ultrasound in the 1970s and magnetic resonance in the 1980s has eclipsed these radiological approaches as physiological measurement tools. Therefore, given tight budgets, ultrasonic and magnetic resonance specialty journals should be preferentially included in many collections today. See the discussion of instrumental journals in the Applied Optics and Acoustics chapter.

Virtually no program of extensive basic physiological measurement or multiple clinical trials is done today without substantial statistical or computing help. Many instruments are essentially run with the help of computer interfaces. Those computers make sense of the signals sent out or reflected by probing beams and help to create models or graphical images to help the researcher visualize what is going on.

The leading journal for statistics as used in clinical trials is Wiley's *Statistics in Medicine.* Topically broader, but of frequent utility are *Biometrika* from Macmillan and *Biometrics* from the Biometric Society.

Journals serving the computerization of physiological monitoring are quite numerous with few clear winners in impact factors. However, there are some useful nuances in underlying subject emphasis that can aid in selection. Academic's *Computers in Biomedical Research* is probably the title that is most intent on intact organism physiology, making sense out of data from a human heart monitor, for example. Its closest competitor in this regard is Pergamon's *Computers in Biology and Medicine.* They are choices one and two in this group.

By contrast, both *Computer Applications in the Biosciences* from IRL Press, and Elsevier's *Computer Methods and Programs in Biomedicine* have a heavily biochemical or pharmacological modelling emphasis. They are less urgent for intact organism physiological monitoring.

An anatomic visualization approach close to more traditional radiology is found in *Computerized Medical Imaging and Graphics* from Pergamon. If the local population of physiologists or clinicians does a great deal of collaborative work with radiologists, this is a recommended methods journal.

# Sciences of the Solid Earth
# and Other Planets

Earth science has developed from one discipline that is academically quite old, geology, and from a number that are relatively more recent: physical geography, limnology and oceanography, meteorology, and even satellite-based planetary astronomy. This essay will primarily concern the more "crusty" parts of the earth, as opposed to its water and atmosphere. It deals with both those earth scientists coming from the in-the-field school of geologists and the planetary modeling school of geophysics, as well as with the many professionals whose interests are a blend of both approaches. Historically, the central disciplinary tension has been between those who study rocks and the forces that led to their regional formations, and those who study the earth and other planets as a whole, or at least, in very large pieces. The former group tends to style itself geologists, and to divide themselves out along disciplines such as mineralogy, petrology, geochemistry, crystallography, and paleontology. A further division among them is among the largely academic "pure" geologists–although they rarely use the word "pure"–and "economic" geologists, a distinguishing phrase that is often used. "Economic" in this sense generally refers to minerals that are financially rewarding. While the popular imagination suggests that these minerals might often mean gems, as a practical matter they generally involve metal ores and fuel deposits. The largest subgroup within economic geology is petroleum geology.

Geophysicists by contrast, tend to pursue topics related to broad

[Haworth co-indexing entry note]: "Sciences of the Solid Earth and Other Planets." Stankus, Tony. Co-published simultaneously in *The Serials Librarian* (The Haworth Press, Inc.) Vol. 27, No. 2/3, 1995, pp. 199-210; and: *Special Format Serials and Issues: Annual Review of . . . , Advances in . . . , Symposia on . . . , Methods in . . .* (ed: Tony Stankus) The Haworth Press, Inc., 1995, pp. 199-210. Single or multiple copies of this article are available from The Haworth Document Delivery Service [1-800-342-9678, 9:00 a.m. - 5:00 p.m. (EST)].

scale phenomena: continent-sized landforms, geomagnetism over time, tectonic plate migration, the earth's deep interior, seismology and vulcanism. For many geophysicists, the air and oceans are an integral part of their planetary vision, and even the geophysical publications mentioned in this solid earth chapter will unavoidably feature some atmospheric and aquatic topics. While geologists tend to study the solid earth for its own sake, geophysicists look to the earth as the closest example of planetary forces in action. Geophysicists fully suspect that similar planetary forces exist to one degree or another on some of the other natural "terrestial-type" satellites of the sun, hence their fascination with space probes to other planets.

There is, of course, much jumping across boundaries: volcanic activity, for example, generates rocks, and conversely the rock and fossil record reveals a great deal of information about the migration and weathering of land masses on planetary surfaces. Over the last two decades the geophysics community has been finding increasing sponsorship from the corporate community. "Explorational" geophysicists have provided tools that help make the earth's thick crust more "transparent" or more readily imaged from the sky in ways that assist "economic" geologists. There is, therefore, some cross-enrollment among societies, particularly in the U.S. Americans can simultaneously belong to the Geological Society of America, the American Geophysical Union, the Society of Economic Geologists, and the Society of Exploration Geophysicists. This is one of the major motivations for seeking out review sources: there can be a number of groups interested in the developments within one of the cognate fields of the solid-earth sciences.

Another motivation for a good review literature is a general division of publishing traditions that needs to be bridged, particularly abroad: one important bloc of scientists is multinational in its publishing habits; the other largely localized. Foreign geophysics journals are generally handled by for-profit firms and have a highly cosmopolitan outlook. Blackwell, for example, handles *Geophysical Journal International* for a consortium of societies: the (British) Royal Astronomical Society, the Deutsche Geophysikalische Gesellschaft, and the European Geophysical Society. Blackwell also manages the lead title of the European Association of Exploration Geophysicists: *Geophysical Prospecting*. This pattern is repeated in titles from a number of the major players in geoscience publishing: Elsevier/Pergamon, Kluwer, and Springer. In sharp contrast to the geophysics situation, where much of the publishing is "internationalized," is the geological pattern. Not only is there an understandable propensity for each country to have an indigenous geological society, but virtually every country, and often the larger states or provinces within a country, tends to have a governmental geological survey office. These offices or surveys, as they are generally called, often publish studies, both "pure" and "economic," pertaining to their jurisdictions. In addition there is a strong history of mineralogical museums in many European countries (and even within some of the larger U.S. academic institutions). Many of these centers also serve as publishers of extensive if irregular museum bulletins, with findings in need of integration into the larger stream of earth science literature.

Of course, some earth science literature is based on phenomena that is not of universal concern but still is of acute interest in several nations. Earthquake-prone parts of the world, most notably Japan, Australia, the Mediterranean, and California, have a commonality of interests and literature issued from seismological stations and, more recently, from facilties for testing earthquake-proof structures. Review sources often incorporate their findings.

## REVIEWS IN GEOSCIENCES

The sciences of the solid earth and other planets are very well served by review papers. *Science* and *Nature* frequently carry reviews of importance to earth scientists, a rarity for most other physical sciences save for, perhaps, sexy astrophysics and particle physics. Reviews of varying styles and lengths are also quite common in the major general-purpose journals of the geoscience community.

*Geotimes,* the semi-popular monthly of the Geological Society of America, offers highly comprehensible tutorial minireviews, a role also played by *Geology Today*, a Blackwell publication issued on behalf of the (British) Geological Society. Longer and mildly more sophisticated tutorials are the special forte of *Earth Science Reviews,* an Elsevier journal which truly fulfills its own advertising claim of "bridging the gap between textbooks and journals of original research papers." A life-and-times minireviews approach is found in the annual awards issue of the *Geological Society of America Bulletin*.

Four journals primarily feature state-of-the-art reviews. Two are hardbounds, the *Annual Review of Earth and Planetary Sciences* from the not-for-profit Annual Reviews, Inc., and the roughly annual *Advances in Geophysics* from Academic. Two are quarterly softbounds, *Reviews of Geophysics* from the American Geophysical Union, and *Surveys in Geophysics* from Kluwer. While the *Advances* consists almost solely of lengthy state-of-the-art papers, it is not uncommon to find at least one life-and-times piece in the *Annual Reviews* or a tutorial in the *Reviews*. *Surveys* features symposia or theme issues from time to time, and also does book reviews.

There are some quasi-review journals as well. The German firm Schweizerbartsche has taken a serial that has a history as an annual, and turned it over time into four more-frequent if still somewhat irregular publications. Thus we have the *Neues Jahrbuch für Geologie und Palaeontologie* and the *Neues Jahrbuch für Mineralogie*. Each has a *Monatshefte* (roughly a monthly) and an *Abhandlungen* (an irregular supplement). The *Abhandlungen* generally have the longest papers, many of a review type. Their style tends to be state-of-the-art although substantial historical detail is often included. *Festschriften*, the quintessential German tribute to older scholars, are also common in the *Abhandlungen*. Both English and German language papers are accepted, although these journals have been slower than most to go largely English.

Among these many sources for reviews, three are very strongly recommended, even for the smallest collections, as follows. The *Annual Reviews* represents the same two things across all disciplines in which it fields an entry: high quality at a low cost. Yet, this particular *Annual Review* is by no means clearly dominant in this discipline. It has roughly equal status with the AGU's *Reviews of Geophysics*, itself a relatively inexpensive title. This is particularly true since it serves as the official organ for the U.S. national reports to the International Geophysical Union. While Earth *Science Reviews* seems disproportionately expensive relative to the other top two, it is also substantially more frequent (8 per year), much better illustrated, voluminous, and it has carved out an educational niche in all decent collections in the field.

This brings us to the second tier. *Advances* is a good fourth choice. While not as readily readable as the Elsevier entry, it is less expensive, and medium-size collections with master's degree students can negotiate its characteristically lengthy papers. *Surveys* is persistently less cited than *Advances*, costs more, and represents perhaps a fifth choice. The *Neues Jahrbuch* family is probably best reserved for the very largest university collections on the doctoral level. Price and lingering language difficulties work against it.

A number of more specialized reviews might be mentioned. Whether they are taken or not is dependent on emphases within given earth science programs. *Ore Geology Reviews* from Elsevier follows the winning format of Elsevier's *Earth Science Reviews* in terms of intermediate length and intermediate difficulty. The primary audience however, is not so much students as college-degreed prospectors and working mining engineers. A more sophisticated approach on the graduate academic level and with a state of the art style can be seen in both *Progress in Physical Geography* and in its companion field, *Remote Sensing Reviews* from Harwood. *Progress* is one of the few earth science serials that also features recurring installment reviews covering advances in designated topics over specified time spans.

Two rather atypical sources of reviews ought to be noted before leaving this section. First, since many geoscientists are rock and mineral collectors, most collections should also take the popular-level *Mineralogical Record*, from a not-for-profit group of the same name. It features a highly informative "Annual World Summary of Mineral Discoveries." In this case, many of the finds are indeed minerals of gem-like quality. Second, a perhaps even more intriguing issuance is the irregular publication of the *Scientific Event Alert Network* hardbound series. This work, sponsored by the Smithsonian Institution, represents a formalizing of the reportage found in the *SEAN Bulletin*, a monthly dealing with earthquakes, tidal waves, volcanic eruptions, massive fires, meteorite impacts, and the like. The format is site-by-site with chronology within site. Overview essays often introduce each section. Reading this encyclopedia-like work is at once enlightening and worrying. Our earth is much more dynamic than one would believe from conventional newspapers in geologically stable areas like New England, although still not quite as exciting and scary as the tabloids everywhere report! It should be noted that somewhat more sophisticated summary calendar reviews are found in professional journals, with the "Summary of Recent Volcanic Activity" within Springer's *Bulletin of Volcanology* a particularly prominent example.

## SYMPOSIA AND THEME JOURNALS IN THE SOLID EARTH SCIENCES

Geologists love to aggregate (there's a pun in there for petrologists) and they cherish the live symposium. No fewer than four broad-interest geology journals, apart from the *Neues Jahrbuch* series mentioned earlier, frequently publish symposia. *Geologische Rundschau* ("geological panorama") from Ferdinand Enke arguably features the most, many of them effectively "festschriften," honoring the life and work of a senior scientist. Many of them, alas, are still in German. The *Journal of the Geological Society of the United Kingdom* generally features three to five papers from regional symposia on a regular basis. They appear, however, alongside other more conventionally contributed papers. This mixed symposia/regular paper format is also seen in *Economic Geology* from the Society of Economic Geologists. When there are symposia with enough papers to justify their own issue, extra copies are made available for later sale. Despite its title, *Reviews in Mineralogy* from the Mineralogical Society of America consists much more often of symposia papers than of extended monographic review essays. While these *Mineralogical Reviews* paperbacks are nominally annual, it is not unusual to see them issued out of chronological sequence, depending on the symposium organizer's skill in obtaining and editing print versions of what typically were oral presentations some time in the past.

Geophysicists appear to have fewer stand-alone symposia series than do geologists, but share in their propensity for special symposia issues of regular journals. Every American collection should have the *Journal of Geophysical Research–Planets*. Despite competition from *Science* and *Nature*, *JGR–Planets* tends to grab most of the papers dealing with the findings of planetary probes and puts them in special theme supplements. In this it beats out other journals of planetary physics such as *Icarus* from Academic and the *Earth, Moon, and Planets* from Kluwer. Kluwer, however, features an irregular hardbound symposium series of longstanding: *Advances in Earth and Planetary Sciences*. Rather expensive, it is nonetheless recommended for comprehensive collections.

A series of regular softbound journals generally fielded by the for-profit sector feature occasional, but important geophysical symposia in a number of geophysical specialties. Including these symposia from time to time is part of a deliberate strategy on the part of their publishers that enables these for-profit journals to compete with some of their less-expensive society rivals in the same topical areas. The four following for-profit series seem to partition the earth into its major structural layers and provide conference coverage of each.

*Physics of the Earth and Planetary Interiors* from Elsevier features both theme and symposia issues, often related to geomagnetism, a phenomenon dependent in part on the internal rotation of the molten cores of planets.

Getting nearer the surface, at the major subterranean plate zones, one finds irregular symposia and themes issues in the *Journal of Structural Geology* from Pergamon/Elsevier and in *Tectonophysics*, another Elsevier title.

For work on the surface, the physical geography segment of geophysics will appreciate the occasional symposia in *Earth Surface Processes and Landforms*, a Wiley title.

Two titles focus on special interests that are not narrowly related to specific geophysical layers. The *Society of Exploration Geophysicists Special Publications Series* is almost always a straightforward symposium publication, dealing with topics of "economic" interest. The mineralogical-geochemical-atmospheric chemical community is well served by occasional symposia in *Geochimica et Cosmochimica Acta*, another Pergamon title.

## *LABORATORY AND FIELD METHODS SERIALS*

Many classically trained geologists focus a good deal of attention on precisely determining the components and structure (typically called the "unit cell") of given minerals, naming those minerals, and then avoiding frivolous renaming or duplicative alternatives to those names. (They have a name authority control attitude that would please even a cataloger!) *American Mineralogist* from the American Mineralogical Society has a section in virtually every issue passing on the validity of new claims. Laboratory analyses of new minerals are key to a number of competing journals. *American Mineralogist* and to a lesser degree the distinguished but now less intensely mineralogical *American Journal of Science* from Yale, are the first choices from the not-for-profit sector. But for most American collections, for-profit titles and foreign competitors are very numerous and very strong. Selection from among their offerings does not appear to be simple.

The British leader is the *Journal of Petrology* from Oxford University Press. The Germans boast *Contributions to Mineralogy and Petrology,* a title now handled by Springer but privately published for decades by Tschermak, a turn of the century mineralogist of tremendous stature. Springer also fields the *Physics and Chemistry of Minerals* on behalf of the International Mineralogical Association. *Geochimica et Cosmochimica Acta* from Pergamon, mentioned earlier as a notable source of symposia, has a genuine mix of U.S. and foreign authors. Despite its off-shore financial backing, it also serves as the manuscript headquarters of the U.S.-based Geochemical Society. *Organic Geochemistry* is another Pergamon title, but this time features a strongly foreign flavor. *Lithos* and *Chemical Geology* are titles from Elsevier with some American participation, but are of an essentially European character. Fortunately amid this maze of "mineralogical," "petrological," "geochemical," and "organic geochemical" titles are some clues that help in sorting out the journals based on historic propensities that still have some validity.

The most conservative or classical "mineralogical" journals tend to stress igneous and the older metamorphic rocks. "Petrology" is a discipline related to mineralogy that is irreverently but not altogether inaccurately referred to as "rock science" by U.S. undergraduates. In simple terms, minerals make up rocks, although over time both the rocks containing the minerals, and the entrapped minerals themselves tend to evolve into somewhat different forms than at the moment of their initial casting (mineralogical metamorphosis).

Journals of the mineralogy-petrology type often have a stress on determining crystallographic structures, often by fairly classical optical means.

The second type of journal, the "geochemical," discusses the chemical elements present in some solid minerals, but often emphasizes the chemical elements present in the air and waters as well. The chemical geologist sees the minerals as part of a cycle of deposition, mingling with fluids, and reactions with the atmosphere. While mineralogists and petrologists tend to focus on regional events that made the rock what it is today, geochemists tend to look at rock analyses as indicators of a broader and more active earth history, which is perhaps more important than the rock itself. Geochemical methodology includes many more laboratory approaches drawn from modern analytical chemistry, including a number based on isotopic and radioactive tracer methods.

A third type of mineralogical journal involves the "organic" geochemical school. Organic geochemists tend to deal with minerals that are remnants of ancient plant or marine life. To a certain degree, organic geochemists are the "wet laboratory" counterparts of the "pick and shovel" paleontologists. Both the newer organic geochemical group and the old paleontological group have been substantially supported by the fuel prospecting and extraction industries. The "organic" in their name comes from the chemical tradition of so designating compounds which feature significant amounts of carbon, which all conventional fuels have in the form of hydrocarbons. The underlying slant of organic geochemists on earth history, then, is often to look for chemical traces of events that suggest promising fuel deposits.

The best representatives of the classical solid "inorganic" tradition tend to be the *American Mineralogist* and the *American Journal of Science*, mentioned earlier, and the following foreign titles: the *Journal of Petrology*, *Contributions to Mineralogy and Petrology*, and the *Physics and Chemistry of Minerals*. The last title, which includes the word "chemistry," might seem somewhat surprising in this group, but its chemistry is much more closely related to the solid state chemistry and physics of crystals than to conventional "wet" chemistry.

*Geochimica et Cosmochimica Acta* leads the geochemistry contingent partly though its outstanding content, and partly through its society ties. It has the broadest range of papers–solid minerals, aquatic and air interactions–of any of the journals in this group. *Chemical Geology* from Elsevier is a good second choice, although it has a more solid-earth emphasis and a more frankly economic tone. A strength with *Chemical Geology* is its stress on isotopic methods, important for dating specimens and tracing their chemical evolution. A number of other journals of atmospheric chemistry mentioned in the air and oceans chapter are worthy of including in collections with a liberal geophysical orientation, particularly for fans of *Geochimica et Cosmochimica Acta*.

*Organic Geochemistry* and *Lithos* are a complementary pair in the carbonaceous category. While both are important for petroleum geology, *Organic Geochemistry* also includes a fair amount of what might be termed ancient biochemistry, while *Lithos* contains a small amount of traditional mineralogy as well. A large number of even more frankly applied journals will be welcome in corporate collections. At the minimum these will most typically include the *AAPG Bulletin from the American Association of Petroleum Geologists*, the *Journal of Sedimentary Petrology* from the Society of Economic Paleontologists and Mineralogists, the *Journal of Petroleum Geology* from Scientific Press, Ltd., and the *International Journal of Coal Geology* from Elsevier.

Three important geoscientific procedures are conducted initially outside the mineralogical lab and involve fairly unique instrumentation. These are borehole drillings, seismic soundings, and remote sensing of the environment from high altitudes. Fortunately, library selection in these fields is somewhat less complicated.

The leader in the more academic concerns in drilling is aptly named *Scientific Drilling* from Springer. Topics covered can include drilling through tundra and glaciers for climatological history, drilling for geological age estimation of various formations on both land and under the sea, and quite simply, techniques and records for ever deeper boreholes. Papers with a more practical concern with drilling can be found in virtually all petroleum engineering journals. One particularly respected publication emanating from the world's leader in drilling technology, Schlumberger-Doll Research, is *Oilfield Review*, a title currently distributed by Elsevier.

Seismology tends to be regarded as always akin to earthquake location and measurement. But this is only the more familiar half of a story of an underground wave phenomenon.

The following is a brief sampler of serials on the commonly understood earthquake side of seismic phenomena. The *Bulletin of the Seismological Society* of America is clearly the professional association leader. It shares the spotlight with a very wide variety of federal and state sponsored publications, some of which are semi-popular but most of which are event-specific technical reports. Among these are *Earthquakes and Volcanoes* (U.S. Geological Survey), the *Monthly Listings of Preliminary Determinations of Epicenters* (U.S. National Earthquake Information Service), and *Seismographic Stations Bulletin* (University of California at Berkeley). There is also a growing contingent of for-profit journals that stress lengthier analysis that is apart from specific seismic events, and that are intended to have greater general applicability. For example, Kluwer's *Earthquake Prediction Research* and Wiley's *Earthquake Engineering and Structural Dynamics* stress precautionary and adaptive aspects of seismic events. Basic studies of tectonic phenomena, which is absolutely fundamental for understanding earthquake seismology, are found in the journals of tectonophysics and structural geology mentioned earlier, and in *Tectonics*, the AGU title, the leader.

What is less well known about seismology is that a tremendous amount of today's exploration geophysics is done through generating shock waves through the ground and looking for discontinuities that suggest faults and pockets (usually of oil or gas). Journals like *Geophysics,* from the Society of Exploration Geophysicists, and *Geophysical Prospecting,* one of several Blackwell publications on behalf of the highly prolific European Association of Exploration Geologists, are filled with seismic studies either alone or in combination with drilling work. Blackwell is launching a new title that makes the link between seismic instruments and subterranean probing even more explicit: the *Journal of Seismic Exploration*. It will complement *Seismic Instruments*, an established but irregular hardbound series from Allerton Press. Two more basic science journals are recommended that may surprise some readers. The *Bulletin of the Seismological Society of America*, the earthquake leader, also contains some exploration work. The *Journal of the Acoustical Society of America,* popularly imagined as having to do with perhaps speech and hearing or architectural acoustics, has long extended its concept of waves to include those used in seismic instrumentation. It might also be recalled that sonar, long used to map the ocean floor, is another acoustic phenomenon covered in this journal.

The literature of other types of remote sensing is covered in some detail in the optics and acoustics chapter. Optical, as opposed to acoustic, means predominate in *Photogrammetric Engineering and Remote Sensing* from the Photogrammetric Society, the *International Journal of Remote Sensing* from Taylor and Francis, and *Remote Sensing of the Environment* from Elsevier. These titles are key to physical geographers, who use them for various visible and infrared lightwave mappings of surface features from high altitude aircraft or from satellites. Radar is becoming powerful enough to penetrate desert sands on earth to find old river beds, and is particularly useful to penetrate the often dense or violent atmospheres of other planets, where visible lightwave probes are frustrated. Variations in the earth's magnetic, gravitational or background electrical fields, and anomalies in the earth's shape and surfaces–the earth is far less smoothly spherical than model globes suggest–are also mapped by "geodetic" scientists through both ground-based and satellite measurements. Geodesy is the special focus of *Manuscripta Geodetica* from Springer, and is a major component of *Journal of Geomagnetism and Geoelectricity,* a Terra publication.

All of these instrumental approaches in the earth sciences–mineralogical determination, seismic probing of the crust, mapping of the surface–have become extremely complicated electronically and conceptually. Three journals serve to aid geoscientists who are neither engineers, computer scientists, nor mathematical modelers by first choice. These are the *IEEE Transactions on Geosciences and Remote Sensing,* and *Computers and Geosciences* from Pergamon, and *Mathematical Geology* from Plenum. Every institution with an active program in the geosciences will need these titles.

# Waves and Images:
# Applied Optics and Acoustics,
# Including Topics in Remote Sensing
# and Medical Physics

Sight and sound are two senses that man has been using to probe his environment for eons. Since the 1800s, scientists have become aware of three relevant factors:

- First, that these senses were based on waves, sound being based on vibrational waves in some medium, light being based on electromagnetic waves capable of penetrating even a vacuum.
- Second, that there were waves of both sound and light that could not be perceived by ordinary means (ultrasound, infrared, ultraviolet, x-ray waves, etc.). Picking up these waves would require new technology.
- Third, that once filtered and focused, waves of both light and sound could become useful probes of objects.

These facts led to three challenges:

- The first was to build instruments to detect and measure these waves when they occurred naturally.

[Haworth co-indexing entry note]: "Waves and Images: Applied Optics and Acoustics, Including Topics in Remote Sensing and Medical Physics." Stankus, Tony. Co-published simultaneously in *The Serials Librarian* (The Haworth Press, Inc.) Vol. 27, No. 2/3, 1995, pp. 211-220; and: *Special Format Serials and Issues: Annual Review of . . . , Advances in . . . , Symposia on . . . , Methods in . . .* (ed: Tony Stankus) The Haworth Press, Inc., 1995, pp. 211-220. Single or multiple copies of this article are available from The Haworth Document Delivery Service [1-800-342-9678, 9:00 a.m. - 5:00 p.m. (EST)].

*211*

- The second was to devise tools that would artificially generate waves at will, and at desired wavelengths or frequencies so as to broadcast or focus them.
- The third challenge was to record the interactions of either sound or light waves with targets, and to interpret the records.


Despite the fact that sound and light waves are different in many aspects, there are also many shared themes. These include wave generation, detection, filtering, and focus. One can store and reproduce images of wave-target interactions. Both types of wave records can be enhanced for clarity. Most importantly, in the twentieth century, optics and acoustics have been tremendously aided by the development of electronics, particularly solid-state microelectronics and computer storage of digitized images. Precise tunability in wave generation, exceptional sensitivity in wave reception, and automated encoding and retrieving of wave-based data have been achieved. We now can "see" formerly invisible gamma rays and focus intense beams of "laser" light with the flip of a switch. We can detect earthquake-like seismic shifts under the ground even when they cannot be normally sensed. Giant submarines without any windows navigate through underwater mountain ranges using sonar. They identify enemy subs for targetting largely through computer retrieval of their opponent's acoustical "noise" or "turbulence" signatures. A satellite may be hundreds of miles up in space and yet detect the relative ripeness of a wheat crop or the spreading of an oil slick because of their respective optical reflectance patterns. We can generate ultrasonic waves we cannot hear but that we can "see" in their interactions with a developing baby within its mother. The last example is symptomatic of a general melding of optical and acoustical instrumentation, linked by electronics, a union that has come to dominate much of today's environmental and medical imaging. An additional enhancement of the relevance of optical knowledge is that many radioactive or accelerated atomic particle beams have a lightwave character and can be focused for probing objects and treating patients. The biomedical engineer and his literature have become full partners in many aspects of the acoustics and optics industries.

## REVIEWS OF OPTICS IN MORE GENERAL JOURNALS AND THOSE APPLYING OPTICAL TECHNOLOGIES

Despite their historic role in pure and applied physics, optics, acoustics, remote sensing and medical physics have not been frequent subjects of many recent reviews in either journals of general science or in journals covering all aspects of physics. The instrumentation generated by these fields is so ubiquitous and reliable that there is a sense of familiarity breeding contempt. There have been exceptions in the past when there was the inception of a striking innovation: lasers and satellite photos in the '50s and '60s, clinical ultrasound in the '60s and '70s, CAT, MRI, and PET scans in hospital settings in the '70s and '80s, the high-altitude tracking of oil spills, volcano plumes, and deforestation in the '90s. Nonetheless incremental improvements, particularly the miniaturization of these wave-based instruments and their coupling with microcomputers with a view towards expert systems, remain an ongoing theme. This ongoing integration has generated many papers in need of correlation.

One finds some reviews in the more general journals of applied physics. The *Journal of Applied Physics* from the American Institute of Physics intermittently carries clusters of thematic reviews with special "R" page numberings. Less formal tutorial reviews involving applicable physics appear in *Contemporary Physics* from Taylor and Francis. But the bulk of reviews come from serials specifically supported by the optics, acoustics, geophysical and physiological measurement communities.

The leader in general optical reviews, by far, is Elsevier's *Progress in Optics*. This is a hardbound, issued at roughly annual intervals, that features very long, state-of-the art surveys. It has dominated the field for over thirty years. The editorship has largely been in the hands of Etienne Wolff, the dean of classical (linear) optics at the leading program in optics, the University of Rochester. Here is a school that has received substantial financial support from the Kodak camera and film people, a case of enlightened self-interest. Enlightened librarians will make *Progress* their first choice.

A softbound quarterly that emphasizes reviews in lasers and the semiconductor electronics that support them is Pergamon's *Prog-*

*ress in Quantum Electronics.* A special emphasis on guided light-waves is found in *Fiber and Integrated Optics* from Taylor and Francis. This source includes a good deal of business discussion in its informal, tutorial-type reviews, an important consideration in a highly commercial technology. These two titles are appropriate for every engineering collection in optics. The remaining optics titles are more specialized.

Large academic collections, and multinational market firms, will want the largely German-language *Jahrbuch für Optik und Feinmechanik* from Schiele and Schoen. Any collection that deals with civilian or military satellite imagery, geosciences, or environmental protection will likely want the *Remote Sensing Yearbook*, a comprehensive hardbound from Taylor and Francis, which deals largely with optical scans and the interpretation of their images.

## REVIEWS OF ACOUSTICS

There is no clearcut leader in the publication of acoustics reviews, largely because there is no journal specifically devoted to them. The largest organization devoted to acoustics publishes the *Journal of the Acoustical Society of America*, but even here reviews are scarce, about three to six per year. There are at least two reasons for this. First, the *Journal* produces a special, technically well-classified bibliography of "References to Contemporary Papers on Acoustics." The society may well regard this as a workable substitute for reviews. Second, as a look at this annual special issue suggests, acoustics is fragmented into many extremely diverse applied specialties. These include speech and hearing, electronic recording and commercial sound broadcast, architectural, mechanical vibrations and industrial noise control, clinical ultrasound, seismological probing, and the largest community of all, underwater sound detection, a militarily critical field still cloaked in much secrecy. Space constraints caused by serving all the original research papers of each constituency seem to preclude extensive special interest reviews for any one of them in this multi-interest journal. Consequently, one is dependent on the occasional review seen in journals of some of these specialties. These include most notably the *IEEE-ASSP Magazine* (tutorials for speech and signal processing), the

*IEEE Journal of Ocean Engineering* (while largely acoustical, also covering underwater magnetism and communication problems), the *Journal of Sound and Vibration* (Academic Press, serving the mechanical vibration and noise control sectors, generally with state-of-the-art reviews) and the *Bulletin of the Seismological Society of America* (an occasional tutorial or state-of-the-art review).

## REVIEWS OF MEDICAL PHYSICS

In contrast to the acoustics community, medical physics, including clinical ultrasonics, is very well served with reviews. These are, however, still widely scattered, and occur in journals devoted primarily to reporting original research papers. Nonetheless, some rules of thumb for finding them are possible. Review writers seem to place their papers as follows:

- When the author is a medical doctor, the reviews appear largely within clinical specialty journals. Thus far the big three have been: obstetrics, cardiology/circulatory, and radiology (a traditional field grounded in x-rays but whose practitioners are in control of other diagnostic and treatment instruments as well). Just as an example, important specialty reviews can be found in the *American Journal of Obstetrics and Gynecology*; *Circulation*; and *Radiology*, and their competitors. Opthalmology, dermatology, and nephrology are seeing more tutorial reviews as laser treatments are used in the eye and on certain skin cancers, while ultrasound is being used to help break up kidney stones. Virtually every surgical specialty now uses lasers to some extent to minimize bleeding during cutting and cauterizing. Most of the reviews in any of these clinical specialties discussed thus far will be of a "consensus of opinion" type, and the discussion will focus on the use of either light or sound waves as either a probe at lower energy or as a kind of curative tool at higher energies.
- A fairly even mix of medical doctors and applied physicists can be found represented in journals devoted to given types of acoustic or optical instrument as opposed to types of organ system or disease. The *Journal of Clinical Ultrasound* from

Wiley and *Ultrasound in Medicine and Biology* from Pergamon are probably the leading source of reviews in a field
crowded with titles. They also provide largely consensus-type
reviews. *Lasers in Surgery and Medicine* from Wiley provides
a somewhat smaller number of reviews for its clientele. *Magnetic Resonance in Medicine* from Academic, and the *Journal
of Computer-Assisted Tomography* are not slanted towards
providing reviews, but offer some background, opinion, and
consensus pieces. Thus far, PET, or Positron Emission Tomography, has not generated its own journal, for reviews, or otherwise.

- Review authors with a background primarily in applied physics dominate two journals with occasional but authoritative
state-of-the-art surveys. These are *Medical Physics* from the
American Institute of Physics, and *Physics in Medicine and
Biology* done by the Institute of Physics for a wide consortium
of societies. These journals also do double duty as leading
sources of methods papers, particularly in beam therapies and
imaging techniques.

There is hope for consolidating some of these disparate groups of
authors into a single journal for reviews. The publication closest to
that goal is *Critical Reviews in Diagnostic Imaging* from CRC
Press, a softbound quarterly with particularly extensive state-of-the
art surveys and matching bibliographies.

## THEME AND SYMPOSIA SERIALS IN OPTICS

Optics is very well served with symposia and theme issues. The
Optical Society of America publishes three major periodicals: the
*Journal of the Optical Society of America A: Optics and Image
Science*, the *Journal of the Optical Society of America B: Optical
Physics*, and *Applied Optics*. Each one issues frequent calls for
papers that match some vital theme, giving manuscript deadlines
and any special qualifications of authors or text. Many of the regularly appearing issues that result are thereby transformed into state-
of-the-art conferences in print. Additionally, a number of actual,
in-person specialized symposia are included as well. Annually,
there is is at least one general OSA conference in optics. It merits a

special convention issue included with subscriptions to these three journals. Each special issue is filled with abstracts of scheduled presentations and some background on the major award winners. The Optical Society of America package belongs in virtually every collection with any interest in optics. Engineering schools will also want the *CLEO* series, the *Conference on Lasers and Electro-Optics* line from the IEEE. Together, the OSA and IEEE entries form the basic core of conference literature.

There are competitors in this field, but most have some *caveats*. These relate less to quality than to problematic collection management.

One famous series that appears almost frenetically is the *Proceedings of the Photo-Optical Instrumentation Engineers*, often cited as the *SPIE Proceedings*. These are generally the camera-ready-copy text of informal programs given across the country by professionals in the optical and electronics industry. It is not unusual to come across over one hundred and fifty new numbers a year! This series is arguably the most up-to-date, if also, because of its strong "workshop" bent, one of the less archively maintained. These are regarded as having a certain ephemeral nature. (If you don't like what you read, wait a minute, there will be a new conference!) It is nonetheless wise for all engineering schools and large corporate electronics centers not only to take, but bind every issue for several years. General purpose academic collections may wish to retain only a few of the more current years.

The for-profit sector provides three worthwhile series that are substantially more enduring in terms of lasting collection value. While they, too, often use camera-ready copy, most are hardbound and marketed for long-term use and as having a broader perspective than the *SPIE* series. The *Springer Series in Optical Sciences* is arguably the quality leader, but a standing order may not be feasible just to get the conference literature it sometime represents. While some of these durable volumes are indeed *festchriften*, conference work or thematic numbers, others are straightforward monographs. This is also true of Plenum's series in *Optical Physics and Engineering*, and Dekker's *Optical Engineering Series*. In all three cases, one must be alert to advertisements or book reviews that indicate that new entries represent collective works.

## SYMPOSIA AND THEME ISSUES IN REMOTE SENSING

Remote sensing conferences are occasionally covered by the leading original reports journals in the field, *Remote Sensing of Environment* (Elsevier) and the *International Journal of Remote Sensing* (Taylor and Francis). Nonetheless, despite its irregular appearance, the *International Geoscience and Remote Sensing Symposia*, frequently referrred to by its acronym, the *IGARSS* series, is the key IEEE publication from the scientific and technical view and should be in any collection with an interest in this field. Various geographical, agronomical, and hydrological society conferences will be of more occasional pertinence. While they certainly use remote sensing techniques, their interest is in the objects being studied rather than in the procedure or tools.

## SYMPOSIA AND THEME ISSUES IN ACOUSTICS

As was the case with its review literature, general acoustics is not as well served as optics in terms of conference and theme literature. Virtually the only conference publications covering all aspects of acoustics are the two meetings special issues produced annually by the *Journal of the Acoustical Society of America*. Their content is almost exclusively abstracts of presentations, however, rather than fully printed talks. Component specialties within acoustics do somewhat better. Many fully reproduced talks are found annually in the *International Conference on Acoustics, Speech, and Signal Processing*, known as the *ICASSP* series from the IEEE. Ocean engineering, including ultrasonics, sonar, and various integrated current, depth, and temperature monitoring systems, is covered in a similar manner by IEEE conferences whose working title changes rather frequently, but can be found by scanning the society's catalog and advertisements under "Ocean Engineering" or the code word *OCEANS*. More occasionally, one finds conference papers or theme issues in the *Journal of Vibration, Acoustics, Stress, and Reliability in Design*, a publication of the American Society for Mechanical Engineering.

## SYMPOSIA AND THEME ISSUES IN MEDICAL PHYSICS

By contrast, applications of acoustics and optics in medicine are frequently accorded conference coverage. Both *Medical Physics* and *Physics in Medicine and Biology* carry meetings papers in some form. The first title always has a special annual meetings issue (abstracts of presentations of the American Association of Physicists in Medicine). The second is more likely to have a selection of fully developed conference papers. Conferences by instrument type are also quite frequent. There is the *Annual Institute of Ultrasound in Medicine Conference Proceedings,* and conference reporting, if not full text, in the *Medical Laser Industry Report,* an important trade publication from Penn Well. Papers relating to either or both acoustics and optics can be found in the broader-based *Proceedings of the Annual Conference of the Alliance for Engineering in Medicine and Biology.* The IEEE sponsors a similar conference series, although, once again, the title is not uniform, and its catalog must be consulted under the heading of "Biomedical." An M.D. authorship is dominant in the bimonthly, thematic issue, Saunders series *Radiological Clinics of North America.* Interestingly, the medical physics titles mentioned earlier carry more papers on strong therapeutic beams, while this radiological series deals largely with the softer beams used for diagnosis. There is yet another association that deals with the hazards of radiation sources or beams: the Health Physics Society. Pergamon handles its journal *Health Physics,* which includes occasional conference papers and meetings abstracts.

## METHODS SERIALS IN OPTICS, ACOUSTICS, REMOTE SENSING, AND MEDICAL PHYSICS

In a very real sense most of the journals discussed thus far could qualify as methods literature. Optics and acoustics are very much "tool" disciplines used by a wide variety of professions and industries. In marked contrast to their relative indifference to the need for reviews and conferences in applied physics, the major English-language physics societies have excellent titles for "tools" journals that frequently have optical and acoustic components. These are the

*Review of Scientific Instruments* from the American Insitute of Physics, and the *Journal of Physics E–Scientific Instruments* from the (British) Institute of Physics. While many of the tools covered have eventual industrial potential, most are described in conjunction with some academic research program. By contrast, a strong manufacturing tone is found in Elsevier's *Optics and Lasers in Engineering* and in Butterworth's Optics and Laser Technology. Like the titles from the physics societies, both are regularly issued softbound titles. The Society of Photo-Optical Instrumentation Engineers, mentioned earlier for its many workshop and informal conference publications, also publishes Optical Engineering, a title very much in line with the Elsevier and Butterworth entries, and its own organization's pragmatic bent.

While an increasing amount of the papers in *Applied Optics*, the OSA title, have involved devices for remote sensing, two other societies offer a more constant involvement. Instrumentation for remote sensing is strongly emphasized in the *IEEE Transactions on Geoscience and Remote Sensing*, while the capture, storage, retrieval, and enhancement of the images (usually from high-altitude aircraft or from space) is stressed in *Photogrammetric Engineering and Remote Sensing* from the American Society of Photogrammetry.

Acoustics remains problematical. It appears to rely largely on a combination of many methods papers in its principal journals, and the issuance of regularly revised editions of standard textbooks/handbooks in acoustics.

Virtually every journal of medical physics, or of a given type of clinical instrument, mentioned thus far contains many methods papers. Nonetheless, a few journals dealing almost exclusively with methods and supporting electronics ought to be mentioned. While the distinction is by no means absolute, the *IEEE Transactions on Medical Imaging* might be regarded as having the best hardware papers, while *Computerized Medical Imaging and Graphics* from Pergamon emphasizes discussion of software and pattern recognition.

# Index

Only the individual journals of which there is significant text discussion are listed; the majority of titles may be found by means of their topic category. Page numbers followed by f indicate figures.

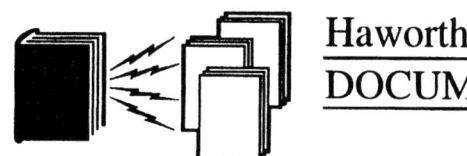

# Haworth
# DOCUMENT DELIVERY
# SERVICE

This valuable service provides a single-article order form for any article from a Haworth journal.

- *Time Saving:* No running around from library to library to find a specific article.
- *Cost Effective:* All costs are kept down to a minimum.
- *Fast Delivery:* Choose from several options, including same-day FAX.
- *No Copyright Hassles:* You will be supplied by the original publisher.
- *Easy Payment:* Choose from several easy payment methods.

---

*Open Accounts Welcome for ...*
- Library Interlibrary Loan Departments
- Library Network/Consortia Wishing to Provide Single-Article Services
- Indexing/Abstracting Services with Single Article Provision Services
- Document Provision Brokers and Freelance Information Service Providers

---

### MAIL or *FAX* THIS ENTIRE ORDER FORM TO:

Haworth Document Delivery Service
The Haworth Press, Inc.
10 Alice Street
Binghamton, NY 13904-1580

or FAX: 1-800-895-0582
or CALL: 1-800-342-9678
9am-5pm EST

---

PLEASE SEND ME PHOTOCOPIES OF THE FOLLOWING SINGLE ARTICLES:

1) Journal Title: _____
   Vol/Issue/Year:_____Starting & Ending Pages:_____
   Article Title:_____

2) Journal Title: _____
   Vol/Issue/Year:_____Starting & Ending Pages:_____
   Article Title:_____

3) Journal Title: _____
   Vol/Issue/Year:_____Starting & Ending Pages:_____
   Article Title:_____

4) Journal Title: _____
   Vol/Issue/Year:_____Starting & Ending Pages:_____
   Article Title:_____

---

**(See other side for Costs and Payment Information)**

*COSTS:* Please figure your cost to order quality copies of an article.
  1. Set-up charge per article: $8.00
                    ($8.00 × number of separate articles)    _____
  2. Photocopying charge for each article:
                    1-10 pages: $1.00    _____

                    11-19 pages: $3.00    _____

                    20-29 pages: $5.00    _____

                    30+ pages: $2.00/10 pages    _____

  3. Flexicover (optional): $2.00/article    _____
  4. Postage & Handling:  US: $1.00 for the first article/
                    $.50 each additional article    _____

                    Federal Express: $25.00    _____

                    Outside US: $2.00 for first article/
                    $.50 each additional article    _____

  5. Same-day FAX service: $.35 per page    _____

                    **GRAND TOTAL:** _____

---

*METHOD OF PAYMENT:* (please check one)
❑ Check enclosed   ❑ Please ship and bill. PO # _____
                    (sorry we can ship and bill to bookstores only! All others must pre-pay)
❑ Charge to my credit card:  ❑ Visa;  ❑ MasterCard;  ❑ Discover;
                    ❑ American Express;

Account Number:_____ Expiration date:_____

Signature: ✗_____

Name: _____ Institution: _____

Address: _____

_____

City: _____ State:_____ Zip:_____

Phone Number: _____ FAX Number: _____

---

## MAIL or *FAX* THIS ENTIRE ORDER FORM TO:

Haworth Document Delivery Service  | **or FAX:** 1-800-895-0582
The Haworth Press, Inc.            | **or CALL:** 1-800-342-9678
10 Alice Street                    |                   9am-5pm EST)
Binghamton, NY 13904-1580          |